HONOURING THE LOSS

HONOURING THE LOSS

A Holistic Guide to Healing with Ritual and Herbal Medicine after an Abortion

Written and illustrated by
India Elyn

AEON

First published in 2022 by
Aeon Books Ltd
Hilltop
Lewes
BN7 3HS

Copyright © 2022 by Elyn

The right of Elyn to be identified as the author of this work has been asserted in accordance with §§ 77 and 78 of the Copyright Design and Patents Act 1988.

All rights reserved. No part of this publication may be reproduced, stored in a retrieval system, or transmitted, in any form or by any means, electronic, mechanical, photocopying, recording, or otherwise, without the prior written permission of the publisher.

British Library Cataloguing in Publication Data

A C.I.P. for this book is available from the British Library

ISBN-13: 9781913504823

Cover Designer: Jessica Coomber

Typeset by Medlar Publishing Solutions Pvt Ltd, India
Printed in Great Britain

www.aeonbooks.co.uk

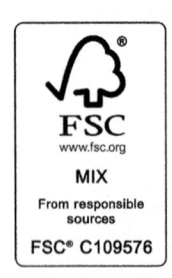

For my grandmothers who stand behind me, and for the women who will one day stand in front of me. I dedicate this book to you.

CONTENTS

DEDICATION — v

PREFACE — ix

CHOICE OF WORDS — xi

HOW TO WORK WITH THE BOOK — xiii

INTRODUCTION — xv

Chapter 1
Herbal medicine — 1

Chapter 2
Before an abortion — 23

Chapter 3
Just after an abortion — 43

Chapter 4

Long term after an abortion   67

Chapter 5

Rituals   85

Chapter 6

Nutrition   115

Chapter 7

Body, movement and voice practices   123

Chapter 8

Boyfriends, partners, husbands   129

Chapter 9

Miscarriage   137

EPILOGUE   *139*

END NOTES   *143*

RESOURCES   *147*

BIBLIOGRAPHY   *151*

GLOSSARY   *153*

ACKNOWLEDGMENTS   *155*

INDEX   *159*

PREFACE

My story

My journey to writing this book has been a long and winding one. It all began high up in the French Pyrenees mountains where I came across a tiny self-published book about abortion and herbs. This discovery sparked a journey of delving into the more ancient uses of herbs for women, as well as exploring the topic of abortion and realising the total lack of resources that exists for women who have gone through one.

When the idea of writing a book about abortion began to form, I had not at that point experienced one, and I had absolutely no intention to, yet life had other plans. Several months later I went through one and felt all the grief and trauma associated with that experience. It took me a long time (and a return to my roots in the UK) before I could sit at my desk and consider writing about this topic. This book is a silver lining to come from that experience. I have lived through one and even though every woman's experience is different, I believe that all women who go through one can share similar threads of their journey. I feel that I made a contract with the little soul who so briefly rested in my womb, a contract to bring abortion out into the open and share with women some of the ways we can heal and be at peace with our decision.

As the months passed I began to feel that I was not writing a book but weaving a tapestry. A tapestry woven with threads of herbal lore, ritual, gentle words, and love. These threads were being woven from many sources by many women; I have not done this alone. Although a book can never replace the presence of a wise elder who is there standing next to you, offering medicine and guidance, as you journey through an abortion. My prayers are woven into every page, so that you do not feel alone in these challenging times. The plants are there to assist you at every stage of the process, even years after, and the rituals are for your soul, opening the door to the sacred in your life and sowing the seed for transformations to occur.

This is the book that I wish I could have held in my hands during and after my abortion. I hope that it finds its way to all the courageous women out there who are called to step on this path of healing and honouring the loss.

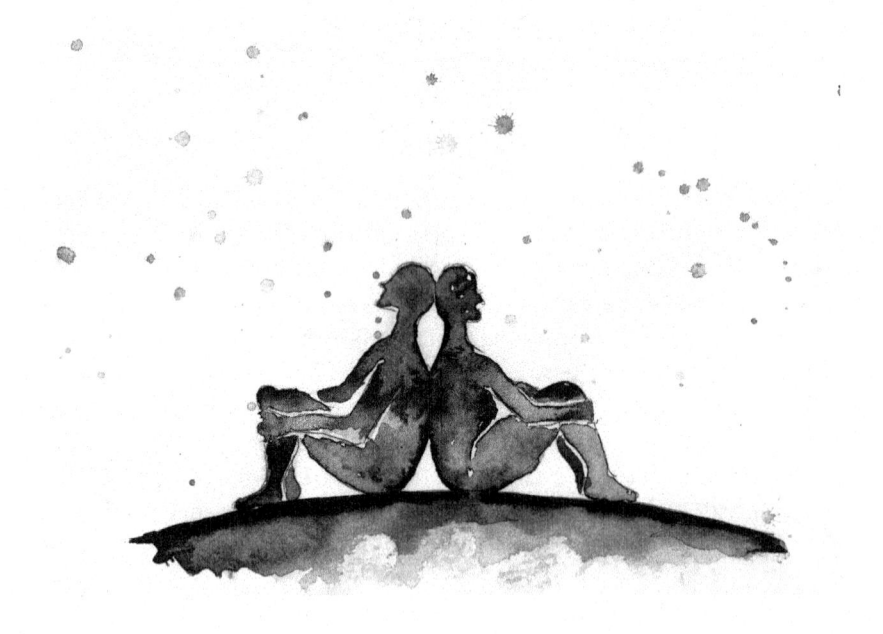

CHOICE OF WORDS

When deciding which word to use for the action of ending a pregnancy, I have chosen the word "abortion". Despite the fact that this word is laced with taboo, politics, and the underworld, it is the one that most clearly represents what a woman is going through. There seems to be no "right" word to use for this extremely sensitive subject, one that is both respectful towards women and is not shrouded in taboo.

However, there are gentler ways to describe having an abortion, such as "pregnancy loss", which can be far less triggering for some women. If you do find yourself triggered by this word throughout the book, then by all means please replace it with words you are more comfortable using.

My choice in using this word was to open up a new space around it, one that is not spoken about and rarely created. This space is one of healing and supporting, which looks beyond how those in power choose to use it. By creating another dimension to the word "abortion", it has the effect of softening the meaning and sound, almost like creating a hidden chamber, one in which only women know how to enter and where there is a place to heal.

I have included the etymology as I have found that looking to the root of the word shows that it is linked to all manner of endings that we encounter in our lives. Sunset being the most beautiful form of ending mentioned. ("sunsets" is not in bold in the original quote)

> Latin abortionem (nominative abortio) 'miscarriage; abortion, procuring of an untimely birth,' noun of action from past-participle stem of aboriri 'to miscarry, be aborted, fail, disappear, pass away,' a compound word used in Latin for deaths, miscarriages, **sunsets**, etc., which according to OED is from ab, here as "amiss" (see ab-), + stem of oriri 'appear, be born, arise'.[1]

What to call "the foetus"?

Another contentious and interchangeable word within the experience of an abortion is what to call the foetus. Each woman seems to have her own way of describing the growing ball of cells within her womb, each perfectly right for her own journey. I have heard many from; "embryo", "the little one", "it", "tiny being", "the soul" , "ball of cells", to no name at all.

Each woman will have her own reason for the name she consciously or unconsciously chooses. This may be dependent on a variety of factors from her belief systems to her desire to connect with the foetus. Another factor may be how far along the pregnancy was, before the abortion took place; as women who end a pregnancy only a few weeks in may have a different relationship to the foetus to those who go through the procedure many weeks later.

Within this book I have thought long and hard about which term to use. In the end I have decided to work with two interchangeably depending on the context. I am using both the "foetus", and "the little being", as I feel that both resonate with the different aspects of the life that was growing in the womb.

If this terminology does not resonate, then just allow whichever word feels best for you to replace the ones that I have chosen.

HOW TO WORK WITH THIS BOOK

Whether you have had an abortion, are considering one, or are simply curious, this book will gently guide you through this journey and beyond, with the help of many healing herbs and simple rituals.

I have separated the book into 3 main chapters;

- The first travels along the journey of the abortion experience, to guide those women who have yet to go through one and are intending to.
- The second is for the hours and days after an abortion, when the experience is still present in both your mind and your body.
- The third is for the months and years after an abortion, where the focus is less on the physical symptoms and more on addressing the emotional side of the experience.

I made this separation of the experience due to different symptoms being present at different times, therefore my suggestions of herbs for that time is unique to that period. However, there are many crossovers, so have a look through all the herbs suggested to see which ones resonate with you and your needs.

I also wanted to open up the possibility for this to be a guide for both women who are choosing to have an abortion imminently and for women who have had one years ago. We are all at different stages of our journey.

I have compiled all the rituals together, so that it is easy for the reader to pick and choose which ones they feel called to. I will specify any that may be more suited to either before or just after an abortion. Woven throughout are recipes and tips of self-care that are there to ease you along this journey. I thoroughly recommend reading through the Herbal Medicine chapter so that you are familiar with the preparations, and how to use the herbs, so that you may use them safely. They are powerful healers and must be treated with full respect.

Please pay attention to any dosages that I give, if in doubt please contact a fully qualified Medical Herbalist for further advice.

Aside from the main chapters, I have included smaller ones on:

- The importance of nutrition for healing the body; how we can nourish our bodies back to balance by including the right vitamins and minerals in our diets.
- Acknowledging the men and the partners who stand by as women go through an abortion. Although many women go through one alone, there are many others who travel through this journey with a partner, who is often left out of the healing equation. He or she is also likely to be affected by the experience, yet can feel at loss about how they can support their loved one through this challenging time.
- Miscarriage. First and foremost a very different experience from abortion. However, many women go through both in their lives and experience similar emotional and physical after effects. I am choosing to acknowledge the similarities within these two experiences, and how all the tools and rituals in this book can be adapted by any woman who has experienced baby loss in her life.

Inclusivity

Although throughout the book I have used the terminology of "women/woman", I acknowledge that there may be people who have had an abortion who identify in other ways. If this is you, please know that this space is for anyone and everyone, regardless of gender, who is seeking to heal from their experience.

INTRODUCTION

Opening the circle

Welcome,

I open this circle of warm smiles and listening ears, a space where women can let go of their burdens and rest knowing that they are supported, free from judgement and held by their sisters. As you journey through these pages and arrive where you feel most comfortable, may you feel heard and honoured for choosing this path of healing. This is not an easy path to step on. But one that follows the moon across the night sky, into the deeper recesses of your soul, then the rising of the sun brings you to a place of peace and acceptance. Take care on this journey. Reach out for support whenever you need, there are always listening ears somewhere and breathe deeply, knowing that you are more worthy of healing than you can ever imagine.

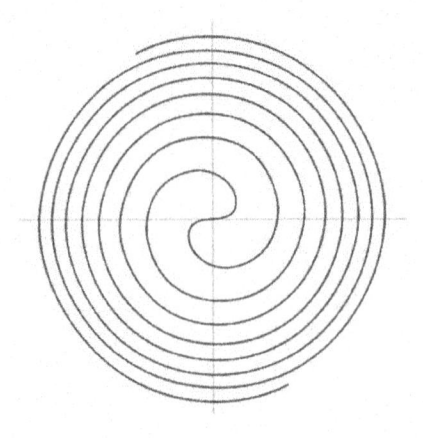

honour is the antidote to shame[2]

The act of honouring is ancient; our indigenous ancestors knew how to honour every aspect of their lives, from the soil they walked on to the deaths of loved ones. Nothing escaped this honouring. Yet how often do we hear this word spoken in today's world? We have similar words such as celebrating, admiring, or appreciating; however, all of those fall at the feet of honour, they do not bear the weight that honour does. Which is why I have chosen it as a doorway into how we can heal from an abortion; in a way that is heart centred, ritual orientated, and sacred. Let us create a new story for women who have had an abortion, one that offers the chance to heal and move through the waves of emotions, and in healing our own stories we create a space for the women around us who may need a helping hand and some kind words. Calling on the strength of ourselves and each other we can collectively as women move forwards, towards a place of peace and acceptance for all we have been through.

Abortion lives in the underworld of our society; despite many women going through at least one, our society still shuns this experience and many countries even refuse to offer this basic right to women. What is the effect of this shaming on women? It means that we must also go underground in our journey, in both having and recovering from one. Women have a history of going underground; this aspect of living sits deep in our bones, we know how to do this, to keep our stories safe and ancient wisdom secret. Yet what goes under must come up. And now is the time that abortion must come to the light. As I look around me more and more women are talking about their experiences openly, there are courses available for women looking to heal, and meditations available for anyone who has experienced baby-loss. This is a sign of positive change and slowly a wider acceptance from our communities.

This book was born out of a deep belief that we as women are allowed to honour our abortion(s) as part of our life's journey. I believe that when we allow ourselves to take the time and space to heal from our experience, we are creating a new story for women and for the generations to come. A story that celebrates the freedom of choice and empowers us to take full responsibility for our healing journey.

This belief has been founded from my own journey with abortion, as well as listening to the many stories from other women who have also experienced one. There was a common thread woven through their tales, a void that existed in the weeks, months, and years that followed. I heard a yearning for support, healing, or a way to honour the loss. As so often happens the resources were not there, so these women, like many others, were left to navigate the often bumpy terrain of the aftermath alone.

Once the abortion is over, we are left standing outside the clinic with a myriad of possible emotions from relief to shock coursing through our veins. As effective as the process of a medical abortion may be, there is very little spoken about regarding after-care. Depending on the clinic and method of abortion, you may receive a small booklet that goes through the physical aspects of what to expect after an abortion, however that is all.

What about the hormones that are running ragged through the body at the sudden change, or the ache in the womb where once there was a small being that has now gone. It is these aspects that I have chosen to acknowledge, I see them as the shadows of the experience, which are easily repressed yet are calling to be transformed into peace and acceptance.

As I moved through the months after my own experience, I began to realise that I wanted to create a space that could offer solace to anyone who has gone through or is approaching an abortion. When I see this space, the invisible world surrounding this book, I see an old kitchen cabinet filled with herbal remedies, a circle of candles gently flickering, each flame representing a little soul that passed through the veil, and an ancient wise woman who represents part of every women, sat in the corner offering her rituals to honour the losses that we all have faced.

Throughout the weaving process of this book I have felt the presence of my own grandmothers and the wise women from centuries gone, who held sacred space for women to cross over the thresholds of life and death. These womb experiences of birth, abortion, miscarriage, death, were treated with absolute respect and reverence. All of life was sacred and valued; these women understood the importance of creating ritual for these transitional moments, and the healing herbs that were woven throughout their work. We all hold this wisdom inside of us, let us return to a place of reverence for ourselves, our wombs, and other women. We are all on this path together.

What does it mean to heal from an abortion?

> "If we are going to find our way out of shame and back to each other, vulnerability is the path and courage is the light. To set down those lists of *what we're supposed to be* is brave. To love ourselves and support each other in the process of becoming real is perhaps the greatest single act of daring greatly."[3]

To heal means to "become whole", to return to the wholeness of your unique self. So by choosing to step on the path of healing after an abortion, you are making the conscious choice to return to a place of balance and harmony in yourself.

Why heal from an abortion?

To heal after an abortion is to address any imbalances that may have occurred as a result of this experience. These imbalances may manifest in either the physical or the emotional, often both. The choice to step on this path of healing is a bold one, particularly in a society that does not recognise the after effects of an abortion as "real". You are paving the way for generations of women to come, showing them that abortion is no "sin"; it is an experience that many women go through in their life, and one that we have every right to honour as a part of our journey as women.

There may be many reasons for a woman to choose to step on the path of healing her experience; but I believe the core of this desire, is a seed of light that is telling her she is worthy of healing. It is like a whisper from spirit to bring up all that has been repressed for generations, summoning it to the surface to be released. There seems to be a collective desire growing among women to no longer ignore the darker shadow sides of having a womb.

One of these aspects is shame, a common feeling when ending a pregnancy. This can be both personal and collective shame; the collective comes from all the other women both past and present who felt unheard and unloved around their abortion. When there is a desire to confront this shame and look straight into its ugly eyes, we begin to unravel ourselves from this complex web of what "we should have done/said/not done/felt". Thus it begins to lose its power over us, as we dig deep into our own stories and pull out the strands of truth from our hearts. In doing so, we become a beacon for all other women, who are seeking another gentler and truer way to honour their abortion.

Ancestral healing

Have you ever asked your mother or grandmother if she had an abortion? It is likely that for women of older generations, going through an abortion was more commonplace due to the lack of contraception available. Furthermore, depending on which country this occurred, the experience is likely to have been very underground, resulting in a potentially harrowing time. Often when talking to older generations about the more challenging aspects of life, we hear how there was less tolerance and acceptance surrounding grief and the outward showing of emotions. This resulted in the suppression of many intense feelings that were maybe never given the space to be released or accepted. When emotions are withheld from their desire to flow through the body, they are then stored within the cells causing an imbalance in the natural flow of energy. This creates a block that can result in a physical manifestation of illness.

We who were born from the womb of our mother, who was born from the womb of our grandmother and so on, can hold all this unexpressed pain, trauma, and grief that these women experienced in their lifetime. If we consciously chose to work through any pain, grief, shame, or trauma that arose from our abortion, we are not only healing ourselves but we are releasing these emotions from all those women that came before us. I cannot testify enough how powerful this is, and what an opportunity we have to send love and blessings down the line of the women who came before us.

Working through generational layers of unexpressed emotion is not a one-step journey, but an endlessly unfolding one, where each time you successfully release one aspect, another will be revealed. As you travel this path, the layers will emerge more readily and the healing will deepen. By engaging on this level of ancestral healing, you are lessening the burden and creating a new blueprint for the future generations of women, see it like wiping a slate clean. During this process, even without sharing your journey with your mother or grandmother, there may be significant shifts within your relationships. This is a sign that you are doing great work and to be patient as you continue gently holding space for yourself.

Changing times

Over the last few years, abortion has been coming to the light, as women begin to realise that this is an experience that must not be buried underground and kept secret for evermore. We have seen this with the recent winning of the right to have a legal abortion in Ireland, campaigns on social media such as #shoutyourabortion, as well as common place discussion of the topic on popular radio shows. There is no denying that abortion is political, this word is laced with legalities, rights and wrongs, and strong opinions. However, I am looking past this side of abortion, to the women who have gone through one and are seeking help, guidance, and healing. This is what matters; how can we move past a place of judgement of each other, into one of true acceptance and grace that we are all here doing the best we can, learning from our experiences and growing along the way.

> I fear that revealing how tough my abortion was gives fuel to those who want to make abortion illegal. I can admit it was tough, and simultaneously know that it was the right thing for me to do at that time. I believe all women should have access to this medical care, and my prayer is that they also have access to the support and love and experience of other women.
>
> —C.G.

Around 1 in 3 women go through an abortion at least once in their lifetime.[4] Abortion is still illegal in many countries and in others its allowed only under certain conditions.[5] This can endanger the lives of the women who choose to have one, as she must find underground ways to go through one or leave the country and seek help elsewhere. This statistic demonstrates how normal abortion is, yet our societies reflect back a very different view on the subject. It is a tragic fact that women are still losing their lives to backstreet abortions, and we can only hope that more governments wake up to the basic human right that is legal abortion.

The womb

The womb is the creative powerhouse sitting deep in our body. This space is where new life is created, and even without the desire to birth a baby, our wombs are always leading us towards a creative and fulfilling life. Although the uterus is the centre of the reproductive systems, it is the ovaries that hold the potential for life. If you no longer have a physical womb, the energy and essence of this space is still fully present in your body.

> Ovarian energy is a woman's creative fire energy. It is the energetic source of life force energy utilised in making children, as well as making any creation a woman brings into the world.[6]

When we are centred in our womb space, we are living our life from a deep and grounded place. We have the capacity to flow effortlessly around obstacles in our path and honour our inherent creativity, whilst balancing the masculine and feminine energies. When our wombs are out of balance, physically or energetically, our whole beings are out of sync. To be clear, a physical imbalance may be a uterus which is sitting in the wrong position within the body, and an energetic imbalance could be a trauma that is still held energetically within the womb space. As the Belizean medicine man Don Elijio says, "a woman's center is her uterus. If a woman's uterus is out of balance, so is she".[7] Unfortunately, this focus on our wombs being an important centre for women is not a widespread belief within our culture; instead it is our minds/brains that are the centre of attention. It is an interesting concept to dwell on for a few moments. If our womb is our centre, then instantly anything that has occurred within our wombs must cause repercussions to our whole self.

For generations past women have had their wombs cut from their awareness, they were simply a place to grow babies. Little was spoken of the "taboo" that was periods, more often called "the curse" (and still are in many cases/cultures). This was the era when women would go to the doctor with symptoms that we could now diagnose as severe premenstrual tension (PMT) and she would be classified as hysterical, mad, and "not right".

When we think of the simple fact that our wombs have the ability to hold, nourish, and birth new life, that in itself is a miracle. However, our relationship to our wombs can quickly turn sour as a result of challenging experiences, such as an abortion. As a result of any pain, shame, or trauma we go through, this cuts us off from our wombs, which consciously or unconsciously severs our relationship to this part of ourselves.

For some women they will never have considered cultivating a relationship with their womb, simply seeing it as just a part of our body. What if we began to create a new kind of connection with our bodies? We would be amazed at what they tell us, and their extraordinary capacity to heal. In turn this would inspire a new level of care and respect for this flesh and bones that we are.

Occurring in our womb space, abortion is amongst the web of reproductive stories that we experience throughout our life as women. Even for those women who feel no need to heal after their experience, there is still a physical imprint upon the body of what happened. The most important aspect is to turn your attention inwards and listen to what your body needs, this will be different for everyone and will vary dramatically depending on all the different elements that were involved in the experience. In these pages I introduce many different ways that you can connect with your womb, from a gentle massage, to creating a womb balm or even having a vagina steam. All these practices are there to help you to create or nourish a connection with this beautiful centre of our bodies.

Cultivating the power to heal ourselves

The freedom to be able to easily choose to have an abortion is one that can leave you feeling empowered. In the UK we are able to freely make that decision, which is a reason to be grateful. However, as the weeks and months pass after the experience, the initial relief of no longer being pregnant may give way to feelings of shame or grief.

When we decide to have an abortion we willingly sign ourselves up for the medical process, putting our bodies into the hands of others, trusting them to stop the pregnancy in the safest way. Once the procedure is complete, either in the clinic or at home depending on the method of abortion, it is then assumed that the experience has ended and we can move on. However, for many women this is not the case. Although the initial feeling could be relief, in the days to come other more painful emotions may surface. In extreme cases, symptoms emerge that are not dissimilar to post-natal depression. Initially we may feel empowered that we have been able to have an abortion, however, as our bodies begin to react to the sudden change, this empowered feeling may be replaced by a feeling of powerlessness.

The word power conjures up a feeling of a dominating (often male) force that exists outside of us, as we live in a world where "power over" others is present and little is spoken about the "power—from—within".

As Earth Activist, Starhawk says "power-from-within is the power of the low, the dark, the earth, the power that arises from our blood, our lives".[8] This refers to the feminine power that back in the history of time; women were initially revered, then later feared for this power that comes from within them. Yet this source of power that we have within is the power of change, transformation, and revolution. True power comes from a heart-centred and grounded place and when we tune in to this force it can impact our lives in a multitude of magnificent ways. As Lucy Pearce, author of Burning Woman writes, "Our power is a natural force, intimately connected to the force of nature, and rooted in our bodies".[9] This power can change the lives of the generations that follow us, as we remember how we are sovereign to that power and it is our right to honour that which is rightly ours. There is a special kind of force that comes from a woman who recognises the power in her body, it is an energy that we are rarely exposed to, yet is becoming more and more common as women begin to take back that power and live their lives from this place of strength.

Irrespective of their abortion experience, each woman holds the power to heal from it. I do not mean you must go shouting from the rooftops, though do so if that is your path in healing. Rather by opening up a space inside of yourself to sit with your experience and allow everything to surface that wishes to, is a small but significant step to carving a new path of acceptance around abortion.

Sharing of our stories

The root of the world courage is "cor", which is Latin for heart. The original meaning of courage was to speak your truth from the heart.[10] If we apply this way of thinking about the word to our lives, we may be able to see how in moments when we were courageous, this strength came from our hearts.

Breaking the silence of an abortion takes courage, courage to step on the path of healing; how many mothers and grandmothers before us weren't allowed to speak up about what they went through. As women we are carrying those ancestral pains, they run through our blood and rest in our wombs. Know that though you carry their pain, you also carry their support. Now is the time to acknowledge that you are worthy of healing from the grief, the pain.

> Opening up about an abortion is a difficult thing to do. But by sharing our stories with those close to us, and by accepting each other without judgment in those moments of radical vulnerability, we can begin to break the silence caused by this painful taboo.[11]

Breaking the silence of an abortion does not necessarily mean in the literal sense of using the voice, it is more subtle than that. Instead it is about women acknowledging the way that this experience affected their lives, how it changed them as women. Who are you since you went through an abortion? It is about casting your mind back to that challenging time and beginning to recognise what it is that you needed then that you were not able to give to yourself. What small act of healing could you do now, after all the time that has passed, that would help soften your thoughts of that experience.

These small acts of recognition may not sound significant, but through the gentle releasing of any pain/shame/anger attached to an abortion, you are bringing in shards of new light into this space of shadow.

Death

We are birthing/dying women[12]

As women we dance the gossamer line between life and death. Our wombs are a sacred space serving as a container for life, a place of nourishment and enormous creativity. Yet woven into that same space of life is the spiral of death, manifested through our periods each month as the uterus sheds her blood. There is no separation between these polarities of life, they are one of the same to be embraced as a whole. This concept in today's world we may find hard to grasp, yet it is one our ancestors took for granted. Within a community there was often a wise-woman who knew the ways of herbs, midwifery, and assisting souls as they left this world to go onto the next. She would be the one to hold ceremonies and rituals for both a birth of a new soul and the death of another, there was fluidity between both and an acceptance of how we as women can have a foot in each realm.

Death is always present in our lives and not always in a form that we may recognise. The earth and the seasons are constantly reflecting back to us the cyclical changes of life, nothing is ever constant. By tuning into to this wisdom of nature, and watching the trees symbolically die each winter to only return bursting with life each spring, we may have small insights into how death is nothing more than a transition. For every death, something new is always born. When considering abortion as a death, we could consider what has transformed in our lives as a result of the experience? This may seem like a big question when caught in a place of grief and could take months or years to emerge, and be different for every woman. However, this insight into how we have changed as women, or how something has shifted in our lives may become an essential key to healing from the experience.

Think of the Dandelion, who despite the odds pushes up through the one crack in the pavement and the desolate waste site where Lilac flowers bloom and Mugwort thrives. This is nature trying to tell us that against all logic, the pulse of life is ever present.

There is no denying that abortion can be an incredibly hard decision to make and carry through with. The nature of women is to create life, whether that is through a physical child or through her way of living; our wombs are our creative centre, which when tapped into has an immense power. So, when we choose to end a life, this decision can be filled with trauma and grief.

> "Through her choice to terminate a pregnancy, the post-abortion woman comes face to face with her abilities to create and destroy."[13]

The Indian goddess Kali is sometimes known as the "essence of Night"[14], she who is both a creator and a destroyer of life, representing the true reality of being a woman. The example that Kali sets is one that our society shies away from, yet when we engage with this shadow side of being a woman, we are taking a step towards reclaiming the power that we are all born with. We are not just the caretakers, mothers, and daughters, but also the ones who are capable of saying "No" to what is no longer serving us. By letting go of all that does not nourish us, whether that is experiences, people, or dreams, we are standing up to our *truth* as fierce and powerful beings. Kali is not the only goddess who can help us see our dark side; the New Moon is another portal into communing with our shadow. With the guidance of this wisdom that is available to us all, we can begin to love and embrace the multi-facetted beings we are.

Types of abortion

There are two types of abortion that most women go through:

1. Medical—this involves taking two pills. The first one is mifepristone, which works by blocking the hormone progesterone, an essential hormone for the womb to maintain the pregnancy. The second one is misoprostol, which makes the womb contract, causing cramps and bleeding as the pregnancy releases from the womb and leaves the body. I refer to this type of abortion as "The Pill Method".
2. Surgical—this involves being under anaesthetic and the use of suction to remove the foetus from the womb.

Throughout the book I shall sometimes refer to the different methods of abortion due to the varying after effects that each one causes. I shall not go into the medical side of them, they are simply there to describe the difference in experiences between the two methods.

The soul

In very brief words, a soul is the eternal essence that is in our every cell, it is an essence that we all have and remains alive in a non-physical form beyond our death. This can be demonstrated by those who are able to connect and tune in with those who died, conveying their messages back to us. When a woman conceives, that moment when the egg and the sperm meet and become one can be seen as the moment a soul enters into a woman's body. However, this is a much debated topic with many varying opinions. Firstly for some people the concept of a soul is too far out in which case this may not be relatable. However, for those who believe that there may be more than just the small growing ball of cells in the womb, I shall talk about the significance of recognising that "other life".

> The spiritual part of a person that some people believe continues to exist in some form after their body has died, or the part of a person that is not physical and experiences deep feelings and emotions.[15]

Why is this relevant to an abortion?

If we choose to recognise that the foetus has a soul, this can bring a layer of comfort to the experience of an abortion. Despite the physical foetus being removed from our body, there is a life that lives on past that experience, in the form of a little spirit. This spirit can be called on and communicated with at any point for the rest of our lives, often remaining near to the mother and acting as a guardian. Some women who have had an abortion believe that when they have children later on in life it is the same soul who has returned to be born again.

This feels relevant to mention because the experience of abortion can take on another level of meaning, if a woman believes that the soul of the tiny being inside of her has not died, only the foetus has. When you believe in a soul, you believe in life being eternal. When we die, it is our soul that moves over to the other side as the physical remains of our bodies remain on Earth. The concept of a soul can bring huge comfort to some women who have experienced an abortion; it can open up avenues to communicate with the soul who so briefly resided in the womb.

From the perspective of a soul, I believe that before we are born, we consciously choose both our parents and the experiences we need to evolve here on earth. Although certain aspects of our life may be seen as predestined, as humans we always have free-will to make our own choices. Within the context of abortion, if there is a soul that would like you to be its mother, and comes in during conception however you choose to end the pregnancy, there is no judgement from that soul. I feel that the soul is entirely respectful of your decision, especially if you have taken the time to communicate why you wish to end the pregnancy. This may not be a widespread belief; however, I am sharing it as a way to broaden the perspective of life and in hope to lighten the load of any women who caught up in the very real space of guilt after an abortion.

Often the most challenging times in our lives are opportunities given to us so that we can grow and evolve. Who knows how the abortion will change you and impact your life, life works in mysterious ways. I am not saying that there is always a silver lining to this experience that is so often fraught with feelings of shame, pain, anger, and regret. Instead, I am opening up another way to see these difficult times in our lives as places to learn, and become even more compassionate and heart-centred beings.

Finally

My hope is for this book to be part of a gentle yet powerful revolution amongst women who are calling on their power and choosing to heal themselves after their abortion. Each time a woman steps on this path, and any path of healing herself, the light of the world becomes stronger. Let us become the beacons of peace and strength we were born to be.

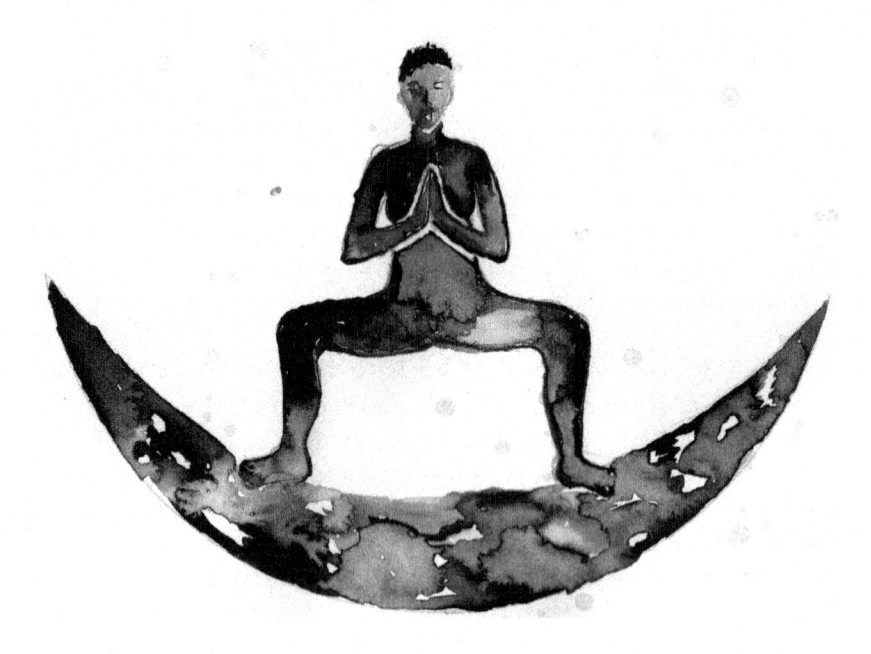

CHAPTER 1

Herbal medicine

Since the beginning of time people have used plants to heal their minds, bodies, and spirits. Every culture on Earth has a history of using their native plants to heal the people and today herbal medicine is one of the most widely used practices, especially in India and China where an unbroken lineage of knowledge has been passed down over thousands of years.

Plants are our ancestors; they have been on Earth for millennia, evolving alongside humans offering their wisdom and medicines for all manner of sickness and disease that we have faced. Herbal medicine honours this ancient knowledge of the plants and as science begins to prove how effective herbs are in healing the body, this form of healing is swiftly becoming more mainstream and accepted within our society.

My journey into the world of herbal medicine truly began when I was travelling around Italy with a tiny backpack and little money. I spent months living with different families in wild and rural locations, helping them on their land in exchange for bed and board. Amongst these families and communities there was often a woman who would go out on the land to gather medicines. My eyes were opened every day to how wild calendula could be gathered to make an oil, or nettles could be transformed into cookies. I soaked up all that I learnt and so the journey began.

Since that time I have been a student to some phenomenal herbal medicine teachers, who have opened the door to the infinite wisdom the plant world has to offer. The plant path is a never ending one of learning and discovery; I delight in sharing their gifts with others and hope that you may too enjoy learning about these wise ones that we share the Earth with.

Herbs and women

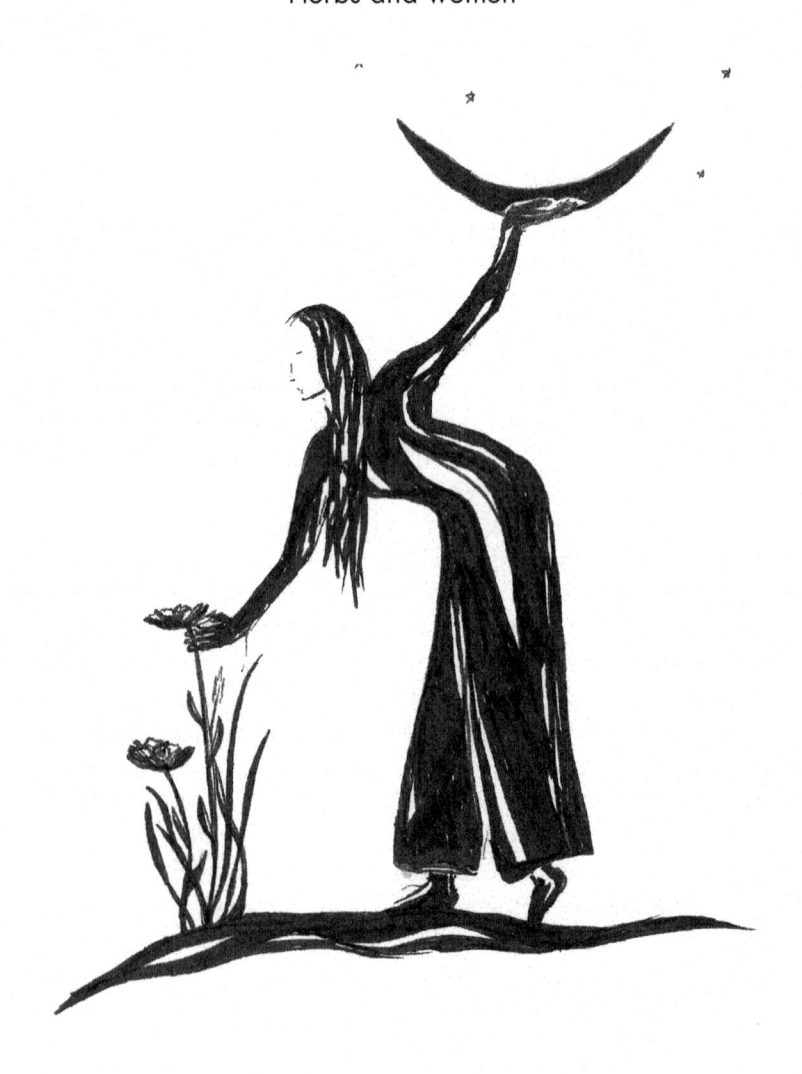

For thousands of years, women have used herbs as a way to control their fertility. Knowledge was passed down over the generations about which herbs to take to have an abortion, control fertility, stop periods, and help the process of birth, to mention a few. These herbs that our ancestors used for the more risky situations, such as inducing abortions and controlling fertility, still thrive here on Earth. The knowledge is held within their leaves, flowers, and roots waiting to be found and put to a healing use again. Often these more specific uses of the herbs can be hard to find, either they are buried deep within old herbal books or are simply exchanged in a passing way from woman to woman. On my travels there have been moments when a gem of wisdom has been shared from one woman to another, often surrounding the theme of how to bring on a late period. These are nuggets of gold, so precious that they almost don't feel real, as if we have suddenly been allowed into an ancient lost lineage of wise women.

In the countries that have legal abortion there is less incentive to look for other ways to go through one, however where abortion is illegal, women are often forced to turn towards herbs. Herbal abortion is an extremely risky undertaking that requires you to go through a very arduous process of consuming a very high (and potentially dangerous) dosage of certain plant medicines. You should be accompanied by someone who has had experience of this process and knows about herbal medicine. Due to the quantity of herbs and duration of the dosage it is very taxing on the physical body and you must know all the warning signs of what could go wrong, with a backup plan to go to a doctor if it does not work. I am in no way advocating herbal abortion, simply sharing a few words about the process. If this is your path, may you find women to support you and be clear with your intention.

Although this book is about how to heal after an abortion, I feel it is important that we are aware that there are plants out there that do have the capacity to end a pregnancy, as much as there are plants the help with fertility to create a pregnancy.

Generally, fear has replaced faith in the way these plants work, yet we must remember that the plants were here a long time before any chemical drug replacement came along. Understandably there can be extra caution when considering using herbal medicine to work with the womb, the powerhouse space within a woman's body that holds the potential for so much life. However, when we work wisely and respectfully with the herbs, we are not only healing ourselves but I believe we are healing that wise-woman lineage that was lost so long ago.

Herbal medicine and pharmaceutical drugs

Today the basis of many pharmaceutical drugs comes from plants. The process begins with isolating a specific chemical in the plant that has been shown to create a positive reaction in the body; this chemical is then combined with various other synthetic compounds to create the drug. Take aspirin, a widely taken pain-killer that contains salicylic acid found predominantly in willow trees. This active chemical constituent was discovered back in the 1920s and extracted to later become a part of the drug that is aspirin. Even though both aspirin and willow bark contain the salicylic acid, they are likely to have varying effects in the body. Willow will not only have the action of reducing pain, but it has other positive effects on the body, such as being anti-inflammatory thus creating a more holistic pain reliever than simply just targeting the pain as aspirin will. This is only one of many examples of how an extract of an entire plant acts quite differently to one that has been isolated within a pharmaceutical drug.

Why use herbal medicine

Choosing to treat your body with herbal medicine can be seen as an act of reclaiming your power and your wisdom. After the clinical experience of an abortion, the simple act of taking a daily herbal tea that you have chosen, can help re-balance your body and create a sense of empowerment that you have the capacity to heal yourself. You have taken the first steps to become responsible for your own health. To be responsible means that we are aware of what it means to be healthy; how can we nourish our minds, bodies, and spirits so that they are in the highest state of health possible?

Herbal medicine is a holistic way to heal the body and bring it back into balance again. Herbs are able to address both the physical and emotional symptoms whilst working on many levels to initiate healing. Although many women will have gone through an abortion, they will not all need the same herb to help them heal. Herbal medicine honours the uniqueness of each and every person, as you will see when looking through the list of herbs that can be used to treat an imbalance, there are many options, and I am leaving it up to your intuition to guide you to pick the herbs that call out to you.

If the concept of trusting your intuition is new to you and you are thinking, how do I know which herbs are right for me? Simply pick one that you like the sound of, it is as simple as that. Begin by drinking it as a tea and notice how your body responds.

Herbal medicine can act much slower on the body than orthodox medicine; the actions of the herbs though powerful can be slow and steady. Although this is not always the case, it is worth mentioning that we live in a world where we can demand everything to happen instantly. Over the counter drugs claim they will remove the symptom within hours, although this may seem miraculous and effective in removing an element of an illness, they are only targeting the surface layer of why you are ill and disregarding the root of the imbalance. If you approach the herbs with a genuine intention to heal, they will guide you back to health and nourish your body on many levels. When taken safely and with respect, there is very little risk of side effects, though it is always sensible to stop taking a herb if you experience any adverse reaction.

There are many other alternative and holistic practices that would be perfectly suitable in helping a woman's body to heal after an abortion. I am focusing only on one; herbal medicine, as this is my passion and I believe whole heartedly that herbs are powerful healers having seem them work on myself and those around me. However, as you learn more about the myriad of ancient healing traditions from around the world and feel called to try others then go for it! They all have their place in healing the people and only by exploring can we feel which ones resonate most with us.

Cultivating a connection to the plants no matter where you live

Today with so many of us living in cities where greenery is kept to a minimum, it can be hard to nurture a connection to nature. Our modern day lifestyle does not lend itself to a life where we can spend the days outside communing with the plants, bees, and birds. Do not let that stop you in choosing to become closer to the natural world. Simply by paying attention to the way that the plants inhabit your landscape can be a great way to learn more about them. You may be surprised by how many plants are able to grow deep within the cracks of cities, demonstrating their will to live and capacity to inhabit our world.

Before I left to go and live in the wilderness of the Pyrenees mountains, I would seek out the wild corners of each city that I lived in. My way of bridging the world of nature and one of urban life was to cultivate a relationship with one special tree, and spend many hours simply sat with my back to this tree. This relationship would be my way out of the intense and hectic pace of city life, and a doorway to a place of peace and connection with the Earth. These experiences taught me that wherever we live, a connection with the soil under our feet and the plants that grow around us is possible, it is simply up to us to find it.

Connecting with the plants

I believe that through consciously opening up to alternative ways to heal our body, we are entering into a new relationship with the Earth. One that our ancestors lived and breathed and one that honours and respects the abundance of life. This is why I encourage you to step outside and connect with the plants and trees. They are longing for loving and respectful connections with us humans. If you are new to the world of herbal medicine, and decide that you would like to begin a relationship with maybe one or several herbs that have helped you heal or you feel intrigued to begin a relationship, here are a few simple steps to take.

How to meet a plant

If you are new to the concept of connecting to the plants, and feel intrigued by this beautiful process then I shall give a few small pointers on what to bear in mind when meeting a plant.

- Decide which plant you would like to meet with. Have you seen it before in the wild? Is it in your local park or the fields around your home?
- Get hold of a good Field Guide and see if you can recognise the plant on your walks. Each plant has its own habitat and some grow in the wild more commonly than others.

Either way, set out with the intention to meet with this particular plant. Initially it can seem overwhelming because there are so many plants to connect with, yet by meeting one at a time you are creating a far more embodied and gradual connection with them.

Once you arrive at your chosen plant, spend a few moments greeting it. This may feel strange, but plants are as alive as you and will appreciate a welcome and introduction of yourself. This begins the connection from a true and heart-centred place. Once you feel like you have made your introductions, start to examine the plant; what are the leaves like?

any flowers blooming? does it have a strong smell? Unless you are 100% sure that it is edible, do not put it in your mouth. All this information from your senses will start to build an image, a story about the plant. If you are familiar with meditation, then you could enter a meditative state, just allowing your energy to merge with that of the plants. This may increase the flow of information you receive about the plants.

If you receive nothing, that is okay, this is only the beginning of your connection with the plant and maybe it will take time to open up. Do not give up.

Drawing or painting the plant is a beautiful way to truly see what is in front of you.

As you do this more often and with other plants, you will begin to notice how differently you feel with different plants/trees. This is a sign you are beginning to allow the exchange of energy to happen and receive information on a subtle level from the plant.

Once you feel like the meeting is over, gently thank this plant. If you feel called to, you may wish to leave a small offering to show your gratitude; this could be a pinch of dried lavender or rose petals.

- One way to continue your relationship with this plant, is if possible, you could try growing it from seed, cultivating a relationship with it throughout its life cycle and maybe even harvesting it for your own teas.

Our ancestors knew which plants to go to when they needed their medicine, long before anyone wrote a book about herbs. These peoples lived in such a close, intimate and respectful relationship with nature that they were able to effortlessly commune with the trees, plants, and flowers around them. Through having such a deep relationship with nature, the plants would communicate with them, allowing these people to gain insight into how to use specific plants to heal ailments and diseases within their community.

Although for many of us there has been a break in this lineage of wisdom, the door to the language of plants is always open to us if we approach them with a true heart and reverence for these green beings we share the Earth with. When we open ourselves up to the world of plants we begin to realise that there is a veritable pharmacy growing right on your doorstep hidden amongst the trees and in the hedgerows. I believe that the potency of herbal medicine is only increased when we make a connection to the living plant. I hope you enjoy your own journey with the herbs.

Working with the herbs in this book

There are hundreds of herbs out there in the world that can be used for every ailment and imbalance. I have chosen only a fraction of these herbs for this book; these are herbs that I work with on a day to day basis and have seen and felt how they can heal the body. Each herbalist has their own favourite plant allies that they work with and you will too as you begin to work with the plants.

I have sought to include herbs that are generally native and/or grow well in the UK. This opens up a door to the potential of creating your own herbal garden and learning what we can sustainably forage from the land around us.

For each herb I include three important elements:

1. **The Latin name**—This is the botanical name for the plant that ensures that everyone is aware of which plant it is. Often plants can have several different common names, so including the Latin name confirms the exact plant species and makes it easily accessible for people from different lands.
2. **Herbal actions**—The way that the herb acts on the body. I am not including *all* of the actions, as the list for some plants is often extensive. If you are interested in finding more out about a plant, I suggest you set off on a path of fascinating research. In the glossary you may find the meaning of all the herbal actions I include.
3. **Plant spirit**—This is the energy of the plant. Beyond the list of medicinal virtues, the plant has a character that makes up part of its gifts. As you ingest this plant you are inviting in these virtues that each plant has to offer.

A large part of my herbal training was about how to connect with the spirit of the plants. I learnt how important it is to honour this side of a plant, in the way that our ancestors did and many indigenous people still do. When I began to recognise that each plant has its own unique set of characteristics and personality, a whole new world of plant wisdom opened up to me. Suddenly the making and taking of herbal medicine becomes much more of a co-creation with the plants. Instead of simply drinking a cup of nettle tea and thinking how it will benefit my liver, you may choose to invite the spirit of nettle into your cup of tea whilst focusing on its qualities of warrior-like strength and fire. By consciously choosing to engage with this level of the plant's intelligence, we are entering into a much deeper relationship with the earth and all her kingdoms.

Herbal preparations

The main preparations are:

- Teas
- Decoctions
- Tinctures
- Oils

Herbal teas

Herbal teas are a simple and creative way to make your own herbal preparations, and an easy way to regularly include herbs into your life. As the herbs mix with the hot water, this draws out many of the nutrients, enzymes, and volatile oils from the plant. Herbal teas are a perfect way to create a moment of calm and stillness in your day, they can become a mini ritual woven into the business of life. As you begin to explore the realm of possibilities with this form of herbal preparation, you will begin to build up a selection of herbs that you really enjoy drinking. Be open to new tastes, some herbs such as Mugwort are very bitter, but over time this taste may be one that you learn to enjoy.

How to make a herbal tea

- Take 1 teaspoon of dried herbs or 1–2 teaspoons of fresh plant material and put into a mug or small teapot (bear in mind that if using fresh herbs you will need to use more than the regular dose).
- Pour over boiling water and cover. Leave for at least 10–15 minutes to allow the water to extract the medicinal properties of the plant. Finally take the cover off, strain the tea, and enjoy your infusion.

At different points in the book I include small recipes for specific herbal tea blends, I use the word "pinch" to describe how much herb to use.

I understand that this is a rough guide, and will vary for everyone. However, it is more for you to experiment with and get to know the tastes of different herbs. You will soon know whether you have put too much or too little of one herb with the taste.

Which herbs to use for a herbal tea?

Most aerial parts of a plant (leaves and flowers) are perfect for a tea. The freedom is yours to choose which herbs you would like to enjoy as a cup of tea, why not experiment with different blends and flavours.

The first step in choosing which herb or herbs you wish to make into a tea is to ask yourself a few questions, this will point you in a clearer direction of which herbs to choose.

- How would you like to feel?
  Calm—energised—nourished—peaceful—balanced
- Are there symptoms in your body that you would like to address?
  Such as: headache—hormonal/teary—lethargic—cramps

How many herbs to put in one cup of tea?

If you have never tasted a herb before then I would advise that you first make a cup of tea with only that herb. This will introduce you to the herb and how it tastes without any surrounding flavours. Once you have an idea of how several herbs taste individually, then you can start blending them. This may take some trial and error, but is a fun and creative process. You cannot go wrong! The worst that will happen is a very bitter tasting tea.

As you become more experienced, you will soon learn which herbs to add to improve a bitter herb and combinations that you grow to love. The bitter taste of herbs can be a new taste for some people, in our diet we don't tend to include many bitter tasting foods, dandelion leaf is a good example. However, bitter often means extremely medicinal with a strong action on the liver. Our tastes evolve over time, so be patient with yourself as your journey this path of herbal teas.

The most important thing is to TRUST YOUR INTUITION, listen to what your body calls for. If that is a new concept for you—then simply see which herb jumps out at you when you read the list. There are now a wide selection of pre-made herbal tea bags available. If you are new to herbal teas these can be a great way to start bringing in the medicinal qualities of the herbs into your diet.

Below is a simple table I have made that lists common symptoms along with just some of the many herbal possibilities that may help in alleviating those symptoms. All of the herbs are quite gentle acting ones, however, if you have any serious health complaints or are on heavy medication then best to consult with a medical herbalist first.

Corresponding herb to symptom table

Complaint	*Herb*
Headache	Lavender Lemon balm Yarrow
Sleepless nights	Passion flower Limeflower Chamomile
Cramps	Ginger Motherwort Sage Yarrow
Irritated/Stressed	Oat straw Lemon balm Rose Chamomile Liquorice
Grief	Rose Lemon balm Tulsi Hawthorn
Depression	Rosemary Lemon verbena Turmeric
Anxiety	Lemon balm Valerian Oat straw Tulsi

Some Herbalists will talk of infusions as well as teas, the only difference is that infusions are teas that are left in the water for a longer period of time, such as overnight. If you are intrigued by the process then give it a go, and discover which way works best for you.

Due to the longer infusion time there will be a greater content of calcium, magnesium, and other minerals present, as well as the medicinal virtues. If you wish to commit to ingesting a lot of one or several herbs over a period of days/weeks then the infusion method can be a useful and easy way to drink medicinal quantities of a herb. Certain herbs lend themselves better to infusions than others, and it is important to note that certain mucilaginous plants are best extracted using a cold water infusion rather than a hot one.

How to make a herbal infusion

Have a large mason/kilner jar ready. If you use a big one such as 32oz one it will mean that you have enough infusion to drink throughout the day without having to prepare another. Put 1oz of plant material into the jar, then fill up with hot water. Place the lid on, and leave to infuse for at least 4 hours. Once you feel that it is ready, strain off and enjoy cool as it is, or you can gently warm it up in pan.

Herbs that work well as an infusion:

– Oat straw
– Nettle
– Lime blossom
– Rose
– Raspberry leaf
– Hawthorn
– Hibiscus
– Damiana
– Red clover
– Marigold

Decoctions

A herbal decoction is the method used to extract the medicinal properties from bark, berries, seeds and roots through a vigorous boiling in water. In order for the active constituents of these parts of the plant to be extracted, they must be boiled in water. This will create a liquid that is much stronger and concentrated than a tea or infusion.

How to make a decoction

Take 1 teaspoon of dried or fresh plant, put into a saucepan and pour over ¾ pint of cold water. Place a lid onto the pan and bring to the boil, then simmer for 10–15 minutes. Allow to cool, strain off the herbs, and enjoy.

Herbs Often Taken as a Decoction

- Dandelion root
- Burdock root
- Hawthorn berries
- Ginger
- Marshmallow
- Yellow dock
- Liquorice

Tinctures

What is a tincture?

A tincture is herbal preparation of a plant that has been extracted in alcohol, vinegar, or glycerine over a period of at least 4–6 weeks. Alcohol is the most popular solvent for making a tincture due to its effective extraction of the medicinal constituents of a plant. However, some people are very sensitive to alcohol so glycerine, which is a sweet liquid derived from vegetable oils, acts as a useful alternative.

Why make a tincture?

Even though tinctures are widely available to buy and are the perfect solution when we really need to take a medicine, we are missing out on the potency and magic of making our own medicines. When we decide to embark on a tincture making mission, this gives us the opportunity to bring intention, love, and prayers into the medicine. Through consciously creating a tincture made with plants that we have chosen, we are making an empowered choice to heal ourselves and connect strongly to one or several plants. Of course there are times when we are unable to make our own, or the need is urgent so we must reach for the ready prepared bottles. However, I encourage you if you have never made your own Tincture to get started by clearing a small place in your kitchen where your little apothecary can begin.

The benefits of a tincture

- Has a shelf life of over a year.
- A concentrated extract of one or several plants.
- An easy and effective way to take herbal medicines, when consuming herbal teas is complicated.
- A simple way to take the very bitter and strong tasting herbs.

How to prepare a tincture

What you need:

- A large glass jar
- Herbs of your choice (dried or fresh)
- Vodka or brandy (at least 60% proof)
- Muslin cloth
- Labels
- Brown bottles
- Your intention

Making the tincture

Take your chosen plants, if using fresh roots make sure they are scrubbed clean of any dirt. Finally chop them up to increase the surface area of maceration.

Place into the clean jar until it is 2/3 full of plant material, then pour in the alcohol until the herbs are completely covered. Place the lid on and *label*.

On the label write the name(s) of the herbs, when you made it, and when you will strain it off.

Store away from bright sunlight, in a cool dark place. Give it a shake every few days for 4–6 weeks. Keep an eye on the level of alcohol as sometimes it can drop, if that happens just top it up so that it is higher than the herbs.

When the time is up, strain off the tincture using a cheesecloth to catch any tiny parts of the plants, and pour using a funnel into a dark brown bottle. Cap and add another label, writing on the date you strained the tincture off, which herbs and alcohol you used and using a word or two, what the tincture is for, i.e. deep peace.

A tincture will last several years if stored in a cool dark place.
Added Extras:

Gratitude

As you go through this process, keep in mind why you are making this medicine. Is it for yourself or someone else? What would you like this tincture to do? What is your intention? Stay present in a place of gratitude for these plants that are giving you their life force. By honouring this process, honouring the plant spirits, we are opening ourselves up to greater gifts that the plants bestow onto us.

The moon

You may feel like harnessing the energies of the waxing and waning moon for your tinctures. Our ancestors were well aware of how the moon's cycle affected everything, from how the plants grew to the tides and even the weather.

Experiment with making a tincture starting on the new moon, leaving it for one and a half moon cycles (around 6 weeks) and straining it off under a full moon. Though subtle, there is certain kind of magic that is present when we work with the ancient rhythms of life and the celestial movements of the skies.

Dosage

Teas/infusions

3 to 4 cups a day is recommended if you wish to see results from the herbs that you are taking. However, if you are just beginning to include herbal teas into your life, then one cup a day is perfectly adequate.

Tinctures

A standard dose is one dropperful (around 20 drops) 3 x a day.

This is a safe dosage for all the plants that I have listed here. Although a medical herbalist will give you a larger dose, this is after a long consultation where they will prescribe herbs specific for your own situation. In the broader case of a book, this dosage is great way to feel how certain herbs affect you. For some very sensitive people the impacts will be immediate. For example, taking 1 dropperful of skullcap tincture 3 x day, could very quickly result in feeling much calmer and peaceful. However, for others the effect may be less. There is no one cure to fix all with herbal medicine; it is a case of tuning into what your body needs and listening to your intuition. The more you can develop individual relationships with plants, seeing how they change and alter your body, the easier it will be to know which ones to take. This is a journey of constant learning and listening.

Infused oils

Infused oils are an easy herbal preparation to make and a wonderful way to bring more herbal wisdom into your daily life. They are a fantastic way to get to know another side of a beloved plant through understanding the effects it may have on your skin not just internally in the body. Once you have grasped the concept of making your own infused oil, you can take it one step further and make your own balms and lotions. The process of making an oil can be a soothing one, and knowing that you are making something for yourself that you can use on your body after an abortion could help you fill empowered knowing that you are taking an active decision to care for yourself. Infused oils can be healing for many parts of the body, however, I am just focusing on oils that are specifically healing for the womb. The process of making an infused oil takes a minimum of 4–6 weeks, so this is something that you can prepare for after an abortion to nourish your pelvic area.

The benefits of using an infused oil

The skin is our biggest organ; anything that is applied to the skin goes straight into the bloodstream affecting our well-being. Applying an oil directly to the skin is a great way to not only topically treat an area but to connect with that part of the body. With an infused oil you have both the medicinal qualities of the oil and the plant that will nourish your skin and body.

When to use an infused oil

A great way to involve an infused oil into your routine is to have a little bottle next to your bed. Before you go to sleep at night is a great moment to put a few drops into your hands and massage your womb/pelvic space. This is a helpful exercise before and after an abortion, though be gentle with yourself as it could be a while before you feel able to connect with that part of your body.

This is also an oil that can be used for a whole body massage, which could be a way to engage with a supportive partner during this journey (if you have one). Often partners, particularly male partners, feel at loss during times when their loved ones are going through pain and grief. By reaching out for a massage from them, which I hope they would gladly give you, can be a way to assist you both to travel this challenging time together.

Infused oils can be made into both balms and creams. I discuss the former later on as a fantastic way to use these medicinal oils and make them into another form of healing skin care.

What you need

A base oil

The base oil is the oil that you will be infusing your plant material into. There are many that you can choose from, each with different properties, however the oils that I list below are ones that have a long shelf life, enabling you to keep your oil for many months.

N.B. Where possible use extra virgin cold pressed organic oils for the highest quantity of beneficial properties.

- Olive oil—provides a high quality base for your infused oil with a high resistance to rancidity and oxidation.
- Sesame oil—a popular oil traditionally used in the East, high in vitamin E and deeply nourishing to the skin.
- Sweet almond oil—a soothing lightly scented oil.
- Sunflower oil—a rich oil high in vitamins A and E.

Fresh or dried?

Dried herbs are a safer option as the moisture has already evaporated from them meaning less chance of the oil going rancid. However, if you have several rose bushes that are dropping their petals and you feel like now is the time to harvest them, like any other fresh plant, leave them to wilt on some paper in a well ventilated space out of direct sunlight for around 12–24 hours. Once they have slightly dried they can then be infused into oil.

Herbs to use

This is an oil to nourish, honour, and re-balance your womb, therefore I'll suggest a few herbs that can do all of the above and more. However, if you feel called to make an oil with one I have not listed here then go for it! The more we tune in to our bodies the more they tell us what they need.

- Roses—for the love.
- Chamomile—brings nourishment, soothing, and gentle fire back to the womb.
- Melissa—lightness and joy.
- Mugwort—connection with the moon.
- Borage—courage, honouring your own power.
- Calendula—has a huge affinity with the pelvic area, soothes irritations and infections and brings strength.
- Lavender—healing on so many levels, connects you with your soul, very relaxing.
- Damiana—an aphrodisiac that honours the return of your sexuality.

How to make an infused oil

There are two main methods:

The Sunlight Method—the long and slow way.

Fill your glass jar ½ to ¾ full with your chosen herbs (if large and leafy you can chop them up). Pour over the base oil ensuring there is at least one inch of oil over the herbs. Fill right up to the top of the jar leaving little space for any air. Tighten the lid well and give it a good shake to make sure that the oil has filled the jar. Label the jar clearly with the type of oil you used, the herbs, the date it was made and when you will strain it. Place the jar in direct sunlight and give it a good shake, infusing the jar with your gratitude for the plants, the oil, and the sunshine.

Leave for 4–6 weeks, giving it a shake every few days.

When done, strain the oil using either a thin sieve or a clean muslin (better for finer plant material) into a clean jar. Re-label. Place in a cool dark area.

The double boiler method—the quick way

Quantities:

It depends how much oil you wish to infuse; a good starting place is—300 ml base oil.

50–75 g dried herbs or 100–50 g fresh.

Take a large saucepan and fill it with a few inches of water. Take a smaller saucepan or heatproof bowl and place your herbs and oil into the bowl. Make sure that the water is not too high up the sides of the bowl. Simmer the water gently for 1–3 hours, keep an eye on the level of water in the pan as it can evaporate quickly. The aim is to gently heat the oil in order to release the medicinal properties of the plants into the oil, if you see the oil becoming too hot, turn the heat down slightly and put a little cold water into the pan. Once the oil is ready, turn the heat off and allow the oil to rest overnight. Once cooled, strain off the oil into a clean container using a fine sieve or muslin. Store in a dark glass jar and label clearly.

This method is useful when you wish to make an oil quickly

A final note on making oils

If this is the first time you have ventured into making your own oils, I hope that you now feel confident in trying out the beautiful process. The only thing that can go wrong is for the oils to go rancid, and it has happened to the best of us.

Try experimenting with different oils, as the same herb in different oils will provide a very different result; for example, rose petals infused in olive oil will smell quite different to being infused in almond oil.

As you journey along this path of making your own healing oils, you may begin to realise that the plants call for the oil that they need. Maybe the idea of mixing calendula with sesame Oil feels strange yet when you think of using olive oil that feels better. There is no right or wrong in this technique, that has been used for millennia as an effective and beneficial way to harness the properties of the plants.

Make your own balm

Making your own balm is a delightful and simple activity to do. Once you have mastered the process, they make wonderful gifts to give away, as well as building up your own medicine cabinet of different balms for a variety of uses. I include a base recipe, one that is easily adaptable to any oils that you may have or essential oils that you wish to include.

This may be an activity you wish to do before your abortion, as a way of preparing your body for what is to come. It is also something that can be made at any other point when you wish to create a little pot of something that will nourish your skin.

How to use a balm

A balm is thicker than a cream, so well suited to smaller points on the body. They can be used for your lips, hands, feet, womb, heart, and any other part of your body that needs some love.

This quantity will make one full 30 ml jar with some left over that you can slather over your body as you please. These jars and other sizes are easily available from many online retailers.

Ingredients:

- 5 g beeswax
- 40 g of good quality olive, sunflower, or almond oil.
  If you have an infused oil that you have already made this is a perfect way to use some.
  Once you have made one jar, you can play around with the consistency, if you wish it to be thicker, then add more beeswax the next time.

To make a womb/heart balm, here is a small suggestion of the oils that would be healing for this purpose. Though as always, trust your intuition on choosing the combination that works for you.

Infused base oils

- Rose
- Chamomile

Essential oils

- Geranium
- Rose

- Frankincense
- Bergamot
- Chamomile

Method

- Gather your ingredients and make sure that the beeswax is either finely cut or in small chunks.
- Prepare a bain-marie, a heatproof bowl resting on a saucepan. In the saucepan add a couple of inches of hot water.
- Turn on the heat to a low temperature, enough for the water to slowly simmer.
- Place the beeswax in the heatproof bowl and stir gently until it melts completely.
- Pour in the oil, it will initially solidify so continue stirring until both the oil and wax are in liquid form.
- Now add a couple of drops of any essential oils (if using). Essential oils are of a potent concentration, so start with a few drops, and add up to 10.
- Whisper your thanks and prayers into the liquid. What would you like the balm to soothe?
- Have your pots ready.
- Pour the liquid from the bowl into a heatproof jug with a spout.
- From the jug slowly pour into the jars.
- Do not move the jars until the balm has set, this may take 20–30 minutes.
- Once set, place the lids on.
- Take a label and write the name of the balm and which oils you included.
- Finally, admire you finished product and feel proud about what you have just made.

CHAPTER 2

Before an abortion

The days and weeks before an abortion are often fraught with intense emotions, not to mention the early pregnancy symptoms of sickness and tiredness. This chapter is filled with herbal medicine, practical ideas, and meditations that you could do to help bring a sense of peace to you and your body during this time. Life could be carrying on as normal, maybe there are children to care for or full time jobs and other responsibilities, yet carving out a small moment each day in the run up to your appointment could dramatically help in the post-abortion period.

The choice whether you wish to connect with the foetus is only yours. There may be many factors determining whether you wish to or not. I am including exercises and visualisations for those women who resonate with the idea and wish to engage in a communication with the little being. You may wish to come back to these exercises months or years afterwards, when the height of the experience has passed over and you are seeking a connection with the one who rested in your body for those weeks or months.

There is no right or wrong way to go through an abortion, each woman's journey is unique and right for her at that time. In the period of time before one, common feelings such as guilt, denial, and shame may be present. This is all normal as it is an incredibly hard decision for any woman to make, and it is not an experience that any woman ever plans to go through, yet many of us do. If you are someone who is about to go through one, then my heart goes out to you; may you have all the support you need around you and remember you are never alone on this journey.

Connecting with the foetus

There is life slowly growing inside of you, a small cluster of cells, which depending on your belief is either with or without a soul. Over the following pages I offer ways to connect with the foetus/little being.

Why communicate with the foetus?

When discussing how to communicate with the foetus I am choosing to use the term "little being", this is to acknowledge that no matter how small that cluster of cells is, there exists something more than the physical.

Walter Makichen was a renowned clairvoyant who specialised in communicating with spirit babies. Women would come and visit him for all manner of reasons surrounding a desire to connect with a baby they lost, or one they wished to conceive. The true stories in his book *Spirit Babies* can open the eyes to how life is much more than we may perceive and helps us to recognise that each soul who chooses to be born, does so for reasons that we may never comprehend.

When talking about abortion from the place of the soul, we may be coming from a belief that we are all here on earth to grow and evolve. We have all consciously chosen our life here, this includes our parents and the challenges that we face. When we bring abortion into this, we can say that the little soul who came and rested in our wombs for those weeks or months chose to only be on earth for that small period of time. The reason that this soul made this choice may be beyond our rational reasoning, it could have been to help us grow from the experience, to initiate us into a new level of bodily awareness or another multitude of reasons.

I am introducing this way of thinking about abortion to open the awareness that life is much more than the flesh and blood we see. For some women, connecting with the spirit of the foetus before an abortion, could help in the feelings of loss afterwards, as the line of communication is open and may help in becoming more at peace with the decision.

> "Communicating with your spirit baby will help both of you clarify and resolve any issues arising from an abortion".[16]

Ways to communicate

Communication could mean anything from placing your hands on your belly to doing a meditation, there are many ways to enter into a dialogue with your inner world. Opening up the path of communication may bring up a lot of grief, so I ask you to approach this journey ever so gently.

From my own experience, I felt this connection to be hugely beneficial in both before the abortion and afterward. It helped me truly acknowledge the loss of my baby and connect with my partner at the time, which then gave him the opportunity to grieve the loss. For some, the idea of communicating with something that you are unable to see may seem strange or even difficult. However, before I begin to explain the process; simply thinking about the spirit of the foetus is opening up the doorway to communication without you even realising it.

A visualisation exercise to say goodbye

Here I offer an inner journey that you can go on to communicate with the spirit of the foetus inside your womb. The intention here is not to bring on an abortion even though you are visualising the process, instead you are creating a connection and by visualising the journey of it leaving your womb, you are preparing it for what is to come and honouring the little life that you are holding.

You can either read through this exercise then continue on your own. Or ask a friend or partner to guide you through the journey. This may bring up a lot of tears so if you are alone, it would be helpful to follow this journey by making a cup of tea and resting quietly for a while.

- Start off by sitting or lying down somewhere that is comfortable. Maybe pull a blanket around yourself.
- Take a few deep breaths to ground yourself in your body and the space around you.

- Place your hands gently on your womb and begin to tune in that space. Ask yourself how does it feel? Are there any sensations coming from there?
- Close your eyes and imagine this golden glow coming from inside your womb, place your attention inside this light filled space. Begin to notice where the foetus is, you may notice other details about it. Remember this little being is not judging you for this decision; it respects your free will. Feel immense love coming from the foetus towards you. In your own way begin to explain what is going to happen, why you are having an abortion, any fears and hopes you have for the experience. How you are feeling about it? Imagine it listening attentively as you speak. Take as long as you need with this dialogue.
- You may wish to say goodbye to it, now see it very gently leaving your womb. Firstly, it detaches from the lining, then ever so gently begins to travel through the cervix until it finally leaves your body.
- Once you have seen it or felt it leaving your body, you can see it either returning to the earth or heading to the sky, to be with the stars.
- With your hands still lightly resting on your womb, take a few deep breaths in and out. Begin to return to the space around you and feel the ground holding you beneath your body.
- Gently open your eyes and give thanks for this journey and opportunity to connect with the spirit of the foetus. You can repeat this exercise as often as you choose before your abortion.

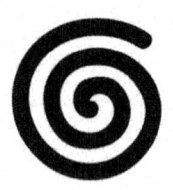

Other ways of connecting

Amongst the pages of a book called *Hygieia*, the author, Jeannine Parvati Baker who was a birth-keeper and midwife has included a testimonial from a woman who was successful in inducing an abortion without intervention. This woman chose to have regular conversations with the "little one", creating a relationship and letting it know that her and her partner had decided that they would like it to leave. Towards the end of her communication, she begins to describe what would happen during an abortion, feeling every last detail until she felt "a sharp twinge of pain" and the next day the blood began to flow.[17]

> "We acknowledged our responsibility in starting life. We had tried to prevent its happening, but it was there. I decided to include that tiny being in the decision of its future. 'Little One', I prayed 'surely you feel our dilemma. We don't want to destroy you, but we feel we can't welcome you joyfully at this time.'"[18]

I have included a summary of this tale as an example of how it is possible to consciously go through an abortion. Although this story may seem exceptional and require a strong sense of visualisation, it is possible. The essence of the tale is that this woman chose to acknowledge that there was another being involved in the conversation, the spirit of the foetus. Through communicating with this being she was able to establish a relationship that would last beyond the experience and provide great comfort in the period of time after.

Although we don't always have a choice about the procedure of an abortion, we always have a choice about how we choose to view it. There are many layers that make up each woman's journey of abortion; not one journey can be compared to another. This uniqueness means that each woman's feelings, emotions, and experiences surrounding the ending of a pregnancy are to be fully accepted and honoured. No one can be the judge of how she is feeling except for her. In the wider reality, a greater acceptance of abortion, creates a more nourishing space for each woman to come to terms with her experience in a non-judgemental and compassionate way.

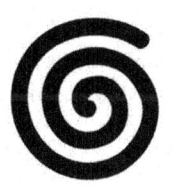

A simple meditation

As the days or weeks pass by before an appointment, your mind may be racing in anticipation/fear/grief of your coming abortion. By taking 5–10 minutes out of your day to sit somewhere quiet and take a few deep breaths will quieten a racing mind and help you to return to your heart and body.

Here is a simple meditation that will help you to be present for a few moments within your day.

If you have never done a meditation before then start by doing only a few minutes, then when you feel more comfortable with the process you can build up from there. If you are finding it hard to switch off then you can accompany this exercise with some calming music.

- Sit or lie somewhere comfortable and quiet, make sure that your back is straight.
- Feel the connection between the floor you are resting on and the solid earth beneath you.
- Feel how the ground is holding your weight completely.
- Close your eyes.
- Begin to take a few deep breaths into your belly, breathe in to the count of 4, pause, then breathe out to the count of 4.
- When your mind begins to race, gently come back to your breath and the rhythm of inhalation and exhalation.
- Continue with this rhythm. If you feel that counting to 4 is not long enough, then begin to count to 5 as you breathe in, and when you breathe out.
- Slowly feel your whole body begin to relax and your shoulders drop down.
- Continue with this rhythm of counting breaths for 10–15 minutes.
- When you are ready to come out, gently open your eyes and return to the space around you.
- Observe how you feel, if there are any differences in your mind or body.
- This exercise can be repeated as many times during the day as you need. Even just a few minutes in the bathroom can make a huge difference.

Practical ways to prepare

Support system

Reaching out to others can be scary, you are showing a vulnerable side of yourself by asking for help when you need it. There could be fear of being judged for having an abortion, so reach out to those that you trust and can offer you the support you need. When thinking about a support system here are a few questions to consider.

- Who is there for you?
- Have you told anyone about the abortion?
- Can someone you trust accompany you to the clinic?

Maybe ask a few friends to come and visit you over the following weeks post-abortion, or to give you a call to see how you are doing. Often people may feel unsure about how to support you best, be clear and honest about your needs. This will provide guidance and better your healing journey. If you feel there is no one in your life who is able to offer non-judgemental support, then there are some fantastic confidential support lines that can offer some much needed support.

I have heard several tales of women wanting to be with and near women during their abortion; it is as if our wombs need the support of other wombs during this time. If you can, try and feel what you need and put those needs first, which can admittedly be hard if you have a lot going on in your life and have a family to look after.

> The next day three of my best girl friends and I went to the country, to the place I call home. I just knew instinctively I needed women around me, and although none of them had been through anything similar, it was a comfort to be with them.
>
> —C.G.

Going alone may be the right choice for you, only you know how you wish to go through this. I hope that this book may give you hope that you are in fact not alone. So many thousands of women go through one, and through being gentle and kind to yourself you are giving yourself the greatest blessing. Each time a woman chooses to acknowledge her decision to end a pregnancy with love, despite what society might say, this is creating a ripple effect that future generations of woman will feel in their bodies and understand that it is only us who have the power over our bodies and only us who are the judges of what is right or wrong in our lives.

Herbs to take before an abortion

The main role of herbs in the days or weeks before an abortion is to encourage a sense of calm within your body and mind. When we are anxious or stressed, our breath becomes shallow and our body tense. By introducing some of the following herbs to your daily routine, these herbs will support your nervous system by strengthening your body's adrenal glands, thus increasing the capacity to cope with this stressful and anxious time. All the nervine herbs can also be taken each evening before bed, if you find yourself unable to sleep.

I have included one extra herb that if you choose to take will begin the opening up of your womb for the abortion. The dosage is very low in the form of a tea; however, it will work on an energetic level to prepare your body.

Nervines

Herbs that are classified as nervines support the body by strengthening the nervous system, reducing the flight or flight response, and returning the body to its natural resting state of being. Some herbs in this category can also enhance moods and ease anxiety. If you are feeling anxious, unable to sleep, or your heart is racing try including one or several of these herbs in your day as either a tea or tincture.

Lemon balm

Latin: *Melissa officinalis*
Herbal actions: Nervine, sedative, carminative, diaphoretic.
Plant Spirit: Dispels states of dark moods and helps bring awareness to the small joys of life again through nourishing the self with love and kindness.

A delightful tasting herb that lightens the mood, brings a greater sense of well-being and joy into life. Particularly good for those feeling nervous and depressed, and also has actions that aid digestion. The lemony taste of this herb is stronger when fresh, however, dried is perfectly suitable as well.

Taken as a tea or tincture.

Oat straw

Latin: *Avena sativa*
Herbal actions: Nourishing, antioxidant, nervine tonic.
Plant spirit: As one of the original Bach flower essences, oat assists in finding one's direction in life after a period of being lost on your path. Oat gently guides you to take new steps towards your dreams in a true and grounded way.

Both the leafy parts and the immature milky seeds are very beneficial to the whole nervous system. The leafy parts are full of essential minerals and vitamins, such as magnesium, iron, calcium, and B-12, making it an excellent choice for a herbal tea.

The other part of the plant that is highly regarded for its medicinal virtues are the milky seeds. These nutritious seeds are harvested as soon as they reach a certain stage and are quickly made into a delicious and nourishing fresh tincture. The way that this plant is able to soothe frazzled nerves and bring calm and peace back into your life makes it an excellent option for restoring the nervous system.

Taken as a tea or tincture.

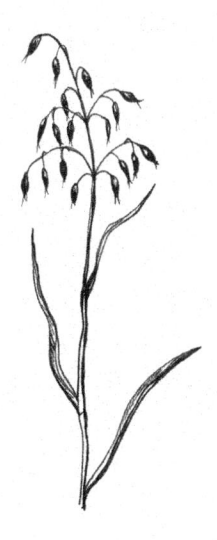

Chamomile

Latin: *Matricaria chamomilla*
Herbal actions: Sedative, carminative, relaxant, antispasmodic.
Plant spirit: These small, cheery flowers of the sun work to nourish the nervous system and help you to feel supported again. Through restoring a gentle strength to the whole self, they will guide you to take the steps you need to find balance.

Chamomile is a beloved herb for helping sleep come easily; these little flowers are also an all-round relaxant that can be taken as a tea throughout the day. As a digestive aid, chamomile can be a useful herb to take if you feel tense during meals, helping you digest your food and relax.

Taken as a tea or tincture.

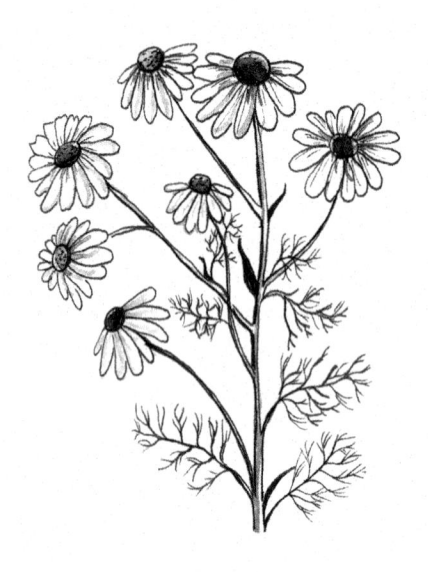

Lime flowers

Latin: *Tilia europaea*
Herbal actions: Nervine, diaphoretic, sedative.
Plant spirit: Encourages awareness in community and the power of cooperation. Welcomes the sweetness of life back again.

Lime flowers are absolute favourites of bees. As they open during the summer months, often you can hear the tree before you see or smell it with its heady sweet scent. These flowers are a gentle nervine and a wonderful sedative taken before bed to aid a restful sleep. Due to their sweet taste they are great to mix in with other more bitter herbs and are very safe to be taken over a long period of time.

A delicious addition to any tea blend though can be taken as a tincture.

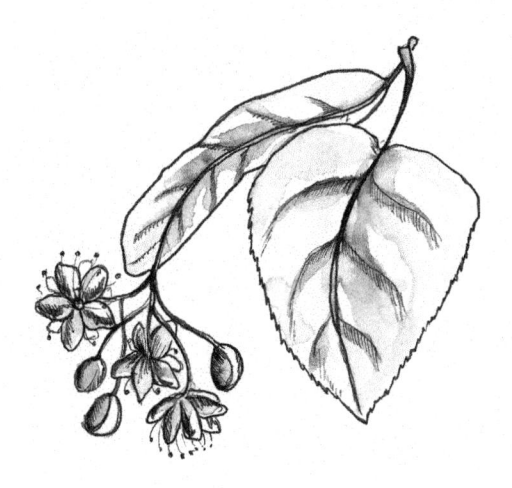

Rose

Latin: *Rosa spp*
Herbal actions: Astringent, sedative, aphrodisiac, anti-depressant.
Plant spirit: Heart healing. Rose offers up her gentle hands of love for anyone going through times of grief and heartbreak. The spirit of rose is able to penetrate deeply into the heart to find that core essence of love, and help bring that love back into one's life.

The way rose can soothe an aching heart, calm the mind, and gently lighten your mood makes it an essential herb to include in your tea before (and after) an abortion. If you can have one ally during this time, rose is the one. She offers up her sweet scent in teas, tinctures, and baths. She will prepare you for any grief that you may be feeling, or trauma that is arising from deep within, asking you to be gentle with yourself and breathe deeply into your heart space.

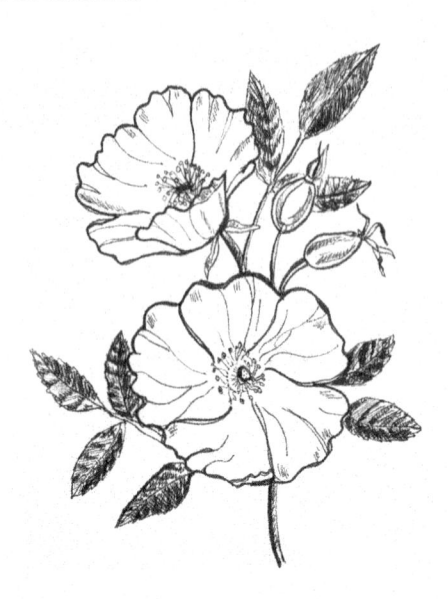

Taken as a tea or tincture.

Passionflower

Latin: *Passiflora incarnata*
Herbal actions: Sedative, nervine, antispasmodic.
Plant spirit: Guides you to become fully grounded so you can open up to higher levels of light from within. Assists with the highest levels of creativity; what needs to emerge after a period of rest?

Passionflower's extraordinary flowers are used along with the leaves to make a very earthy tasting medicine. The principle use of this herb is to nourish the nervous system, helping reduce any tension and restlessness in the mind and body. This is also a useful herb to take before bed if you have trouble sleeping.

Taken as a tea or tincture.

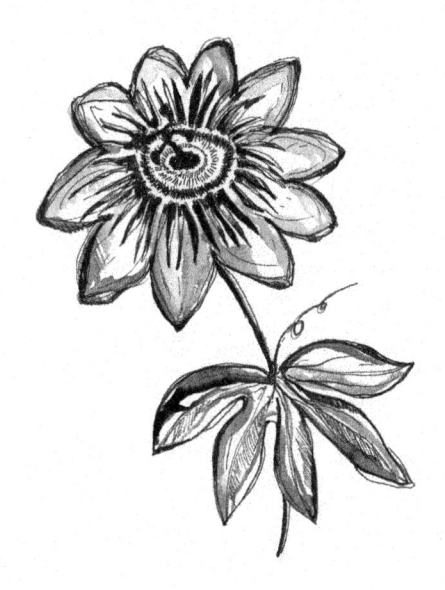

Skullcap

Latin: *Scutellaria lateriflora*
Herbal actions: Nervine, antispasmodic, sedative.
Plant spirit: Skullcap grounds nervous and scattered energy with her essence of calm. Especially useful for extra sensitive people who feel everything very deeply, she helps us to reveal and speak our truth and create from a balanced place.

Skullcap is a widely used herb for nervous tension and stress, even though it is a sedative it doesn't make you sleepy like some of the other herbs in this category. It can help ease muscle tension and headaches as well as soothing any irritability that you may be feeling.
Taken as a tea or tincture.

Morning sickness

Morning sickness can be debilitating, by including one or several of these herbs as teas into your daily routine may take the edge off any nausea you are experiencing and help ease you through this temporary period of time before an abortion.

Ginger

Latin: *Zingiber officinalis*
Herbal actions: Anti-inflammatory, anti-spasmodic, carminative, antiseptic
Plant spirit: Alights the fire in your belly, bringing life back to your body after feeling withdrawn from life. Draws attention to your inner flame, is it burning bright?

The warming and spicy ginger root is a useful remedy for any nausea related issue, whether that is vomiting, morning sickness, or travel sickness. Simply grate a thumb size of the fresh root into a mug and pour hot water over the top to make a tea. To make a stronger infusion, once you have grated the root, put it in a pan with a large mug of water, bring to the boil, once boiling turn down the heat and leave to simmer for around 15 minutes before drinking. Due to its anti-spasmodic properties, Ginger can also bring relief if you experience menstrual cramps, therefore it would be a useful ally to take throughout the abortion. Seeing how readily available and popular ginger is I would recommend taking it as a tea, if you suddenly feel a wave of nausea come out of nowhere and you like ginger, then I have had success with simply eating a couple of slices from the root, which makes for a fiery snack! The tincture can also be taken.

Basil

Latin: *Ocimum basilicum*
Herbal actions: Sedative, antispasmodic, carminative.
Plant spirit: Helps transform any guilt or shame held in the body, especially within the womb space. It is a powerful purifier within the body and energy fields, cleansing away any disempowering feelings.

Basil has a long tradition as a soothing and calming herb, by reducing nervous irritability and bringing clarity back into the mind. A naturally cooling herb that is useful in headaches as well as relieving moments of morning sickness during early pregnancy. A couple of fresh basil leaves crushed in hot water and drunk as a tea makes a delicious drink. In the summer you may wish to try "Sun Tea", where you fill a glass bottle with cool water and a couple of fresh cooling herbs, such as basil, melissa or mint. Leave for a few hours in the sunshine, then enjoy this light tasting and refreshing drink.

Peppermint

Latin: *Mentha x piperita*
Herbal actions: Carminative, diaphoretic, nervine, antispasmodic.
Plant spirit: Clears the mind by restoring clarity to thoughts, helpful in decision making. Through gaining more clarity, the path forward can become clearer.

A refreshing tasting herb that is well loved as an after-dinner herbal tea. In the case of morning sickness, especially in warmer months, peppermint's cooling taste can help take the edge of any nausea and provide relief to the stomach. If you find yourself enjoying the taste of peppermint, why not try growing it in a little pot. The flowers are beautiful and you will always have some mint medicine on hand whenever you need it.

Preparing the womb for an abortion

I am including this small section for those women who would like an ally to help them connect with their womb before an abortion.

Mugwort

Latin: *Artemis vulgaris*
Herbal actions: Emmenagogue, diaphoretic, nervine.
Plant spirit: Guides you across thresholds, removes any blocks in your path, and assists the dream time and how the dream is integrated in life. Nourishes the feminine energy within and allows it to flow freely through life.

Beautiful mugwort has such a strong affinity with women that it is worth mentioning her role before an abortion. I am suggesting that you include a pinch of the dried herb in any herbal teas that you make in the weeks or days before your appointment. Although one of her actions is to bring on a period, this small dose is unlikely to do that, rather you are asking her to open up your womb therefore preparing it for what is to come.

This is more of an energetic way of working with the plants, as you are calling on their vast intelligence and asking them to be involved in your healing journey beyond just the physical.

I once heard a saying about mugwort from a Spanish friend:

"If every woman knew how powerful mugwort it is, she would attach a branch to her jacket every day".

What if you start bleeding before the appointment?

There exists a scenario whereby your body spontaneously decides to have an abortion before your appointment at the clinic. This is a far from rare occurrence as once the appointment has been made with the date in the diary, you are telling your body that you have made that commitment to have an abortion. This could be the moment when the foetus understands that you are committed to this decision, and decides to depart your body without intervention. Technically this is called a miscarriage, as there has been no intervention, however sometimes the line is thin between these two forms of pregnancy loss.

If you suddenly discover that you are bleeding, then I would phone up the clinic to tell them and they will talk you through what to do and what to look out for. This may be a case of just allowing the body to go through the process unaided. However, if you feel like you are bleeding very heavily then it is very important to call for medical help or go and see a doctor and let them know what is happening.

Some fears may arise such as whether the entirety of the foetus/placenta will come out, and what will the foetus look like. This is all perfectly normal, and your clinic should be more than happy to talk to you about these possibilities. It is VERY important to look out for excessive bleeding, if you are soaking through more than 2 pads in 30 minutes then that is a sign that you must seek IMMEDIATE MEDICAL ATTENTION. There are likely to be several large clots, all dependant on how many weeks pregnant you were, so it could look like a heavy period.

Practical ways to soothe your body
Flower baths

Flower baths—An ancient bathing ritual involving water and fresh or dried flowers that help cleanse the spirit and uplift a soul.

Spiritual bathing has been around for millennia across the many cultures in the world where water was recognised as a sacred carrier of life that could cleanse and purify the body, mind, and spirit. By creating a sacred space involving water, prayer, and flowers the impact of emotions such as grief, trauma, and anger can become less, as you choose to allow some of these feelings to be washed away in the water.

Flower baths are strongly connected with the Mayan and Inca ancient healing practices; traditional healers would commonly make a flower bath for a patient that had suffered trauma/grief in their lives and was in need of spiritual healing. The element of prayer is crucial to this ritual, through the power of chanting, singing, or speaking, the water becomes infused with your intention, turning the water and flowers into a sacred vessel of healing.

> The sacred spiritual bath always includes water and prayer, and sometimes flowers and plants.[19]

Prayer is a broad term and often deemed exclusive to certain religions, however it is simply a way to communicate with the spiritual aspect of life using words that resonate with you; there is neither a set way to pray nor a set amount of words to say. Depending on your own culture, family traditions, religions, and beliefs, you can create your own prayers that have true meaning to you. The most important aspect of any prayer is that your words are a sincere and honest expression coming from your heart.

When to have a flower bath

There are an infinite number of reasons to take a flower bath, here are just a few:

Before an abortion—A flower bath could be a beautiful way to soothe an anxious mind and spend some moments alone in a peaceful space.

After an abortion—Taking a flower bath afterwards may help heal any trauma or grief that is felt. On the other hand, if your overwhelming feeling is one of relief you could take one in celebration of your body and the return back to "normal".

Which Flowers/Plants to Use:

Where possible gather fresh herbs and flowers, if not then dried ones are perfectly good. If you are able to go foraging but are not too sure which flowers grow nearby, take a reputable Wild Flower Guide with you and you may able find the following (be sure to gather responsibly and from a clean chemical free environment):

- Elderflowers
- Dandelion flowers
- Burdock
- Primrose
- St. John's wort
- Wild rose

Flowers and herbs you may find in your garden:

- Rosemary
- Thyme
- Marigolds
- Rose
- Comfrey
- Hyssop
- Lady's mantle
- Motherwort
- Sage
- Basil
- Mint

As you set off to gather your flowers and herbs, hold the intention of why you are having a flower bath strongly in your mind and ask to be shown which ones would like to be gathered, this will lead you to the flowers/herbs that wish to be part of this beautiful ritual.

When you are gathering your bouquet of chosen flowers it is important to whisper words of gratitude and blessings; thank them for the life force that has created such colourful abundant blooms, thank them for willingly giving themselves over to your flower bath . Through entering into this place of gratitude you are showering the Earth with loving feelings of reciprocity, that will be returned to you ten-fold as you bathe in water filled with blessed flowers and herbs.

*** *A Prayer to the Plants* ***

Mother Earth, Father Sun, Elementals of this land, I give thanks to the spirit of this plant for allowing me to gather their flowers and leaves and for bringing their healing gifts to my body and soul during this Flower Bath. Blessed Be.

How to have a flower bath

The first step is to gather a good handful of flowers and herbs as spoken about above. Fill a bucket, or washing up basin with clean cold water and place the plants in the water. With your hands slowly start to massage the plants in the water, helping them to break down and infuse the water with their healing properties. This is a good time to say your prayers to the water, state your intention for this flower bath: how would you like to feel? what shifts would you like to take place in your inner being?

Breathe in the aromas of the plants mixing with the water. Once you feel that the plant matter is readily mixed together with the water, leave to infuse outside in the sun if possible, if not then somewhere warm and dry for several hours. For ease you can make this preparation 12 hours before, so that you are ready to take a bath in the morning.

Once the flower water is ready you can choose which kind of flower bath you wish to take:

- Outside—On a hot summer's day this can be a refreshing and exhilarating way to take in the healing properties of the flowers and herbs. If you wish you can involve someone you trust to help you. Take a chair and place it in a sunny spot, somewhere quiet and private. Strip down to how little clothing you feel comfortable in or a bathing suit. Dip a cup into the flower water and begin to pour it over your head, allowing the petals and leaves to cascade over your body. This can be a beautiful ritual to do between two people. As the water falls over you, allow it to dry naturally in the sun, you will look like you have emerged from deep within the earth. Take a moment to sit with the ritual and give thanks for all who participated.
- In the shower—Carry a little stool or chair into the shower, if you feel the flower water is too cold then add some hot water to the bucket. Once comfortable, begin to pour it gently over yourself, breathing in the aromas and sensations as the petals and leaves fall over your body. To avoid blocking the drain, place a strainer on the drain. If

you are warm enough allow the water to fully dry on your body before towelling off.
- Inside bath—Run a bath to the temperature that you desire, you could make the space extra special with a few candles around or some incense burning. Pour the flower water into the bath, if you prefer strain off the plants before pouring the water into the bath. However, it is a joyful experience to bathe surrounded by flowers and leaves. Soak for around 20–30 minutes, taking the time to breathe deeply, meditate, and enjoy the stillness around you.

CHAPTER 3

Just after an abortion

In this chapter I shall talk through the hours and days following an abortion. This period of time after the experience can be tough, as any feelings of relief can be quickly replaced by ones of sadness, guilt, or shame. There may be a rawness to your days, as hormones attempt to rebalance and you try to return to a certain normality. Anything and everything can be accepted in these hours and days; your emotions may swing from one extreme to the other as you begin to integrate everything that just happened. The whole experience may seem hazy as "the availability, speed and comparative ease of the medical procedure belies the reality of what is taking place".[20] It could be weeks or months before you are able to cast your mind back to what you experienced when the pregnancy ended.

Often the initial days are rooted in the physical, as the body is the primary guide. It is not until the body has begun to rebalance that the psyche has space to tend to any wounds from the experience. The environment of a medical abortion does not make you aware of the potential disruption an abortion can cause to your emotions and spirit. However, when we approach healing with the mindset that everything is interlinked, from our womb to our heart and to our soul, then a web starts to emerge, calling in parts of ourselves that need some gentle care in the weeks and months after an abortion.

> A woman's entire being is potentially aligned with the womb of the earth through her sacred phases of menstruation, lovemaking, pregnancy, birthing and menopause. Whenever any of these innate phases is unnaturally disrupted, waves of disturbance and shock reverberate through her vagina, her ovaries, her psyche, her womb, her heart.[21]

My guidance is to be gentle with yourself, if you haven't told anybody about the experience then those around will expect everything to be the same, so it is very important to have that bath or take a day off work, to give you and your body the time to process everything on your own terms.

This is a time to seek support from those around you if possible, having someone there to give you hugs, or simply listen will make the world of difference. Certain things could become triggering; such as seeing babies, talking to pregnant friends, or even being with your own children. Establishing boundaries during this time is also important; because abortion is rarely acknowledged as the significant and traumatic time that it often is, this can mean that people's reaction towards it can be rather brusque. Only share your experience with those you trust to be non-judgemental towards you. It may seem like the outside world is carrying on as normal, yet you feel different in yourself and your body and may find it hard to connect with what is going on in your life. This is a sign from your body to rest; you have just been through a major life altering experience. In some cases, women may continue to bleed several weeks after their abortion, this is another way the body is trying to communicate to take it easy during this time.

Below is a list of symptoms to be aware of if you have taken the abortions pill(s). It is likely that you will have received similar information from the clinic, but I am also including this comprehensive list with kind permission from the team at Clue, who have a wealth of knowledge on all things female.

Is everything okay? Possible complications

It's common to wonder if everything is okay while or after experiencing an abortion. In most cases, there is nothing serious to worry about. Here are the things to look out for after your abortion:

Symptoms that signal a possible complication:

- A fever of lasting more than 24 hours
- Heavy bleeding that doesn't stop, or soaking more than 2 sanitary pads per hour, two hours (or more) in a row
- Worsening pelvic pain in the days following the abortion
- Continued symptoms of pregnancy after 2–4 weeks
- Absence of a period after 8 weeks
- Bad-smelling vaginal discharge
- Minimal or no bleeding in a medication abortion, paired with continued pregnancy symptoms.

If you experience any of these things, contact your healthcare provider. They may be a sign of an incomplete abortion requiring more treatment, or of an infection. Infections can happen when not all tissue is expelled during the abortion.

Severe pain with or without bleeding may be a sign of an ectopic pregnancy (a pregnancy that is developing outside of the uterus, usually in the fallopian tube). Abortion procedures are not treatments for ectopic pregnancies, as the pregnancy will continue to grow. An ectopic pregnancy must be treated as a medical emergency.[22]

From my own experience I wanted to rest, sleep, and recover. I felt like I had had a brief initiation into motherhood, yet one that I decided to cut short in hope for it to return another time, a better time. I had the distinct feeling of waking up feeling different the next morning, a transition had happened, something had passed through the liminal space between life and death. I felt this sudden and deep connection with all women across time who had lost babies, especially those women who had come before me. Within the grief there was a sense of being held, I was not living a new story.

I drew strength from these women who had been there and felt the same emotions, the pain and loss. In those moments I made a vow to my womb who had endured this hardship that I would forever be thankful for every period that came after, for her returning cycle and seasons. Though I didn't know it yet, having an abortion would deepen my connection with my cycle and my body, creating more respect and life for this physical form.

Leave in Beauty

May you hold
yourself in love,
for your body,
your womb
and the little being that has departed,
Call down the stars,
The sun,
The moon to ease this
passing.
As the Earth,
turns,
The cycles of life and death
turn too,
Go in beauty,
You sacred, blessed being.

Herbs

There are several groups of herbs that can help begin to rebalance and heal the body as soon as you have had an abortion. The first thing to consider is how is your body? Check in and notice, Are you bleeding heavily? Are there aches or cramps? Is there tension in other parts of your body? Maybe there are no physical symptoms, only emotional ones such as a heavy heart or teariness. By taking a moment to notice what is going on, this will give you an indication of which herbs your body needs and lead you to choose ones that resonate with how you are feeling.

As with all the herbal suggestions in the book, there will be many variables about which ones you choose to use depending on what you have growing around you or have easy access to. I will specify if there is a herb that is generally best taken in tincture form, otherwise all the others are perfect as singular herbal teas or used as part of a blend.

Below is a list of possible symptoms that your body may be going through and some of the suitable herbs to take. I am not including a comprehensive list of all possible herbs, as there are so many to choose, so I am including only the ones that I would use, each herbalist has their favourites. If you are interested in getting a tailor made herbal prescription, then it would be advisable to book an appointment with a qualified medical herbalist.

Heavy bleeding

NB. A note to classify *heavy bleeding*; if you have taken the two-pill method to have an abortion, then you may have what seems like a heavy period with a few more large clots than normal, though this can vary for every woman. The aim with taking herbal medicines isn't to stem the flow, as the body is reacting normally and is letting go of the foetus and the lining of the womb. With any abortion there is a risk of haemorrhaging, if you are in any doubt after the abortion that you are bleeding an excessive amount then I urge you to phone the clinic or a doctor and ask for medical advice.

Nettle

Latin: *Urtica dioica*
Herbal actions: Astringent, diuretic, alterative.
Plant spirit: Nettle is the plant of the warrior, bringing strength and vitality in times of weakened states of being.

Nettles are high in many essential minerals, such as iron and magnesium as well as vitamin C, A, and K, so it's a brilliant herb to take (and sustainably harvest in spring) if you are bleeding a lot, as they will replenish your body with the iron that is being lost through the blood. Nettle stimulates the liver, cleansing the body of toxins and waste; this is an important action after an abortion, particularly following the ingestion of pharmaceutical drugs, to support their metabolism and excretion from your system.

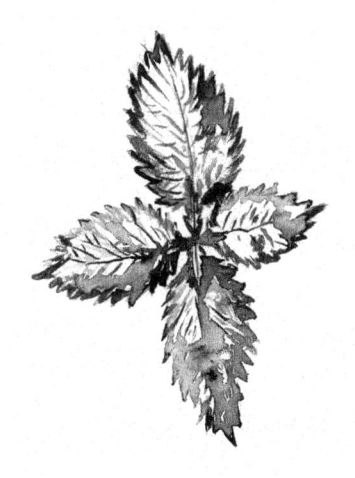

Yarrow

Latin: *Achillea millefolium*
Herbal actions: Astringent, styptic, alterative, diuretic.
Plant spirit: Yarrow helps to strengthen boundaries with those around you and your environment and protect from unwanted energies.

One of yarrow's well known virtues is its ability to staunch the flow of blood. Being both styptic and astringent means that whilst it can be applied straight onto a wound, when taken as a hot herbal tea it can dramatically reduce the flow of blood. Post-abortion when we are likely to feel vulnerable and open, yarrow is there to offer up her presence and help you feel safe and protected.

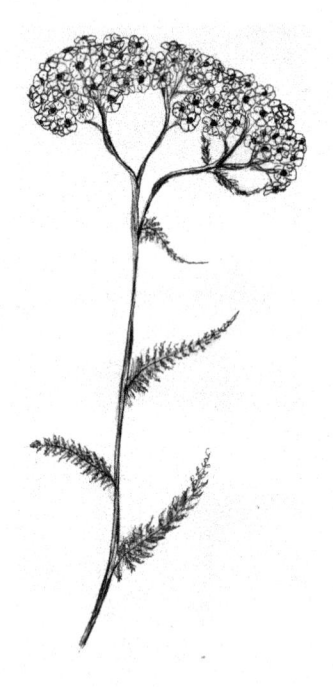

Raspberry leaf

Latin: *Rubus idaeus*
Herbal actions: Astringent, a pregnancy tonic.

Plant spirit: Nurtures kindness and compassion with yourself and others. Helps you take steps to nourish your life and appreciate its fruits.

Raspberry leaf is a helpful herb with a strong affinity to the pelvic area of women. Much loved for its long traditional use of toning and strengthening the womb before childbirth, raspberry leaves can be taken as a way to restore general health of the womb, as well as helping to moderate blood flow due to its astringent properties. High in vitamins and minerals, this herb can be taken over a long period of time following an abortion as a tea or tincture.

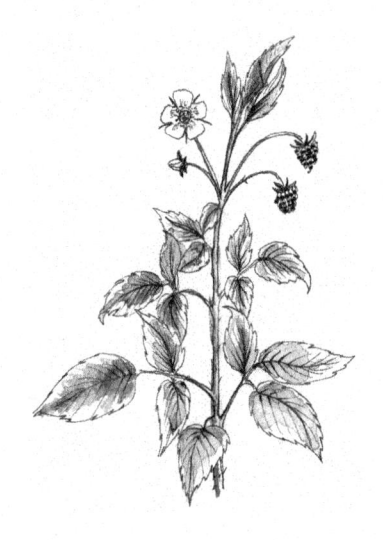

Rose

Latin: *Rosa spp.*
Herbal actions: Astringent, sedative, aphrodisiac, antidepressant.
Plant spirit: Heart healing. Rose's gentle hands of love work deeply on the energetic level of the heart. She is always there to assist in times of grief and heartbreak, bringing softness back into your centre.

Rose heals on many levels after an abortion; in the case of bleeding the flowers' astringent properties will help to moderate excess blood flow, and as a tonic aids the uterus so that it may return to full health. Rose can be taken safely as a tea or tincture.

Lady's mantle

Latin: *Alchemilla vulgaris*
Herbal actions: Astringent, anti-haemorrhagic, styptic.
Plant spirit: Supports and holds women as they go through challenging times. Restores self-worth and rebalances both the heart and womb space.

Lady's mantle is highly regarded as a herb that can curb excessive menstrual bleeding. The astringent properties come from the high level of tannins in the herb, which staunch blood flow and assist in the healing of any wounds. Lady's mantle is extremely safe and would make a useful addition to any herbal tea that you are taking after an abortion. A great combination to aid in the rebalancing of the womb would be lady's mantle, raspberry leaf and rose.

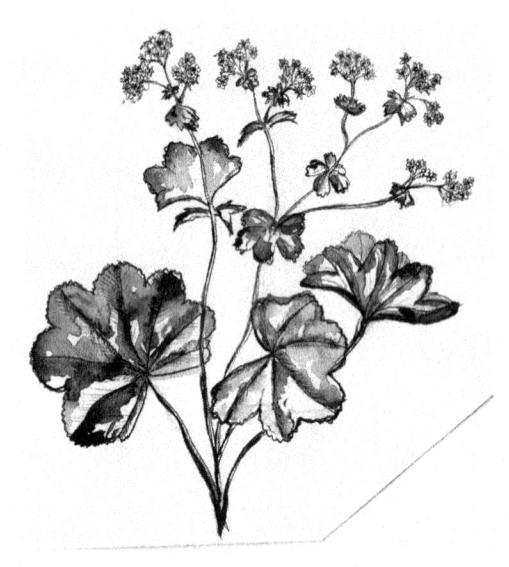

Shepherd's purse

Latin: *Capsella bursa-pastoris*
Herbal actions: Strongly astringent, diuretic, anti-haemorrhagic.
Plant spirit: Helps you to acknowledge your own strength and wisdom, nourishes the heart and womb connection, and allows you to feel held and supported by life. Brings blessings from the wise woman who lives inside of all of us.

This delicate looking plant has a long history of being used by midwives and wise women in the birthing room to stop and prevent haemorrhaging. This is due to its highly astringent properties and vitamin K content, which encourages the clotting of blood.

If you are someone who usually has very heavy periods and are concerned that after an abortion there may be significant blood loss, then having a bottle of shepherd's purse tincture nearby could be a good idea. If in doubt about dosage, consult a medical herbalist for further advice. If you are lucky enough to have the living plant growing nearby, then it would be a great idea to prepare it for after the abortion; make a litre of herbal infusion from the fresh plant, so that in the case of very heavy bleeding you can take regular sips of the tea.

Cramps

Ginger

Latin: *Zingiber officinalis*
Herbal actions: : Anti-inflammatory, antispasmodic, carminative, antiseptic
Plant spirit: Alights the fire in your belly, bringing life back to your body after feeling withdrawn from life. Draws attention to your inner flame, is it burning bright?

Due to the hot and heating nature of this root, ginger works by relaxing muscle tensions. If you are experiencing cramps and feeling cold or shivery then ginger is the one for you. Simply grate a thumb size of the fresh root into a mug and pour hot water over the top to make a tea. To make a stronger infusion, once you have grated the root, put it in a pan with a large mug of water, bring to the boil, once boiling turn down the heat and leave to simmer for around 15 minutes before drinking.

Cramp bark

Latin: *Viburnum opulus*
Herbal actions: Antispasmodic, sedative, astringent, uterine tonic.
Plant spirit: Balances the duality of life. Helps integrate both sides of life, the shadow and the light. Brings in harmony.

Cramp bark as its name suggests reduces uterine cramps and muscular tensions by relaxing the muscles of the uterus. Best taken as tincture or a decoction due to the bark needing a longer time to draw out its properties. Refer to the chapter on Herbal Medicine to see how to make a decoction of the bark.

Motherwort

Latin: *Leonurus cardiaca*
Herbal actions: Sedative, nervine, antispasmodic, cardiotonic.
Plant spirit: Awakens a fierce desire to speak your truth and stand your ground. She asks: are you connected to your line of female ancestors? what are you carrying forward from this mother line? Helps you to let go of that which no longer serves, so you may shine as a woman.

Motherwort is here for the women of the world, a lion-hearted plant that relaxes muscles making it useful for cramps and tensions held in the womb. This plant soothes the nervous system without the side effect of sleepiness, easing tensions and irritability. Best taken as a tea or a tincture.

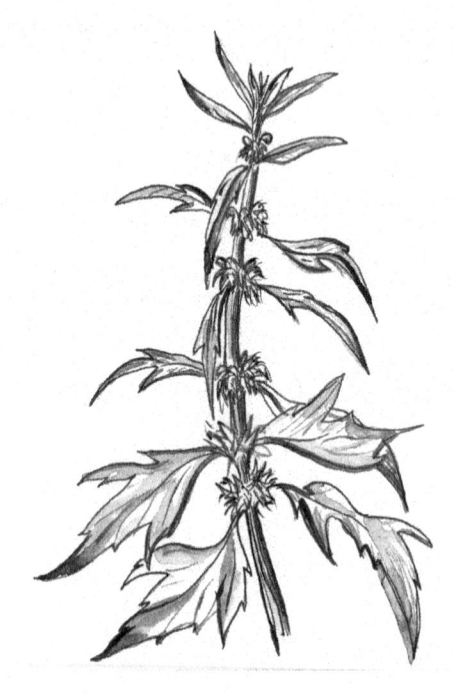

Catmint

Latin: *Nepeta cataria*
Herbal actions: Antispasmodic, sedative, nervine, carminative.
Plant spirit: Catmint grounds and calms, invite her in during times of nervous tension and scattered energy when you wish to return to the root back into your body.

Combining the action of soothing tension and providing light relief from cramps, catmint makes a wonderful addition to any tea after an abortion. Although primarily used as a nervine for restless children, this potent herb works equally well on adults, especially in cases of nervous headaches. Taken as a tea or tincture, due to volatile constituents, be sure to cover your mug once made so as not let the aromatic oils evaporate.

Anxiety/depression/grief

Anxiety, depression, and grief are all distinct and very difficult states to be in, that can manifest in a multitude of ways depending on each person's experience. The reason that I have included them under one heading is that many of the plants can help to address more than one of these difficult states of being.

A note on these symptoms—All the herbs I list below are for mild to moderate symptoms of anxiety, depression, and grief. If you are suffering from severe symptoms, then it is important to seek professional help.

Oat straw

Latin: *Avena sativa*
Herbal actions: Nourishing, antioxidant, nervine tonic.
Plant spirit: As one of the Bach flower essences, oat assists in finding one's direction in life after a period of being lost on your path. Oat gently guides you to take new steps towards your dreams.

Nourishing, balancing, and replenishing in both tea form, and as the milky oat seed tincture. Oat straw tea is a fantastic way to include many minerals into your body thanks to high quantities of calcium and magnesium, which will all help you heal after an abortion. The delicious tasting milky oat seed tincture is a very useful and soothing medicine that can help balance frazzled nerves and swinging emotions. Tea made from the oat straw is an ideal tonic tea to make in a large batch in the morning, so that it can be drunk freely throughout the day. Works well combined with raspberry leaf and melissa as an all-round nourishing herbal tea.

Rose

Latin: *Rosa spp.*
Herbal actions: Astringent, sedative, aphrodisiac, antidepressant.
Plant spirit: Heart healing. Rose offers up her gentle hands of love for anyone going through times of grief and heartbreak. The spirit of rose is able to penetrate deeply into the heart to find that core essence of love and help bring that love back into one's life.

Strengthens the heart, soothes the nervous system, and softens the harder edges of grief. An all-round gentle tonic that can be easily mixed with any other herbal tea, and taken over a long period of time. If you have any wild roses growing near you, such as dog rose (*Rosa canina*), why not gently collect a few of the petals to add to your teas. *Rosa rugosa* with her huge rosy hips is another highly medicinal wild rose that you may be growing nearby.

Skullcap

Latin: *Scutellaria lateriflora*
Herbal actions: Nervine, antispasmodic, sedative.
Plant spirit: Skullcap grounds nervous and scattered energy with her essence of calm. Especially useful for extra-sensitive people who feel everything very deeply. She helps us to reveal and speak our truth and create from a balanced place.

Skullcap eases anxiety, supports letting go of worries, and helps to welcome sleep. This delicate little plant makes a very grounding and nourishing cup of tea. Especially suited for those who have a restless mind and feel agitated by life. Can be taken as either a tea or tincture.

Lemon balm

Latin: *Melissa officinalis*
Herbal actions: Nervine, sedative, carminative, diaphoretic.
Plant spirit: Dispels states of dark moods and helps bring awareness to the small joys of life again through nourishing the self with love and kindness.

A delightful tasting herb that lightens the mood and brings a greater sense of well-being and joy into life. Particularly good for those feeling nervous and depressed, and also has actions that aid digestion. The lemony taste of this herb is stronger when fresh, however dried is perfectly suitable as well.

Taken as a tea or tincture.

Lemon verbena

Latin: *Aloysia citrodora*
Herbal actions: Sedative, antispasmodic, nervine, carminative.
Plant spirit: Helps us to recognise the small joys in our life. Nurtures a connection to the stars. Brings light to parts of the self that are hidden, and gently reveals these parts so that they can be transformed.

A delicious tasting lemony herb that can increase the appetite and help with digestion. Lemon verbena is also a gentle sedative and mood enhancer that soothes and reinvigorates the whole system. This herb is great taken as a tea throughout the day when feeling low or before bed to aid sleep. Can also be taken as a tincture.

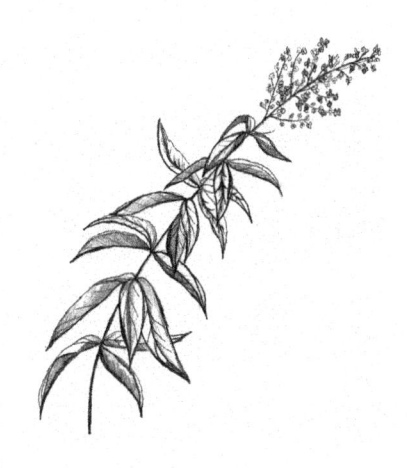

Motherwort

Latin: *Leonurus cardiaca*
Herbal actions: Sedative, nervine, antispasmodic, cardiotonic.
Plant spirit: Awakens a fierce desire to speak your truth and stand your ground. She asks: are you connected to your line of female ancestors? what are you carrying forward from this mother line? Helps you to let go of that which no longer serves so you may shine as a woman.

As well as her virtues that I mentioned above, motherwort is a cardiac remedy easing heart palpitations and tensions, all of which could be associated with grief and anxiety. Makes a great addition to a herbal tea blend that includes lemon balm and rose. Taken as a tea or tincture.

Tusli

Latin: *Ocimum sanctum*
Herbal actions: Adaptogen, antibacterial, antidepressant, antioxidant.
Plant spirit: Tulsi carries a huge amount of light, which she pours into anyone who asks. She helps realign you to the essence of your soul.

Tulsi, a native and sacred plant to India, is generally used as an adaptogenic herb (an versatile tonic and balancer) to increase general health and reduce side effects from stress. Tulsi will restore energy levels in the body whilst clearing away any mental fog. Easily taken as a regular tea or tincture.

Liquorice root

Latin: *Glycyrrhiza glabra*
Herbal actions: Adrenal restorative, antiviral, demulcent.
Plant spirit: A soother in spirit as much as she is in herb form. Wraps a gentle blanket around you so that you may take all the time you need to restore your strength after trauma or illness. Increases levels of patience and tolerance with yourself and those around you.

Liquorice root tastes quite different from those liquorice sweets that you may have tried. An extremely sweet tasting herb, liquorice is known to soothe and heal in all its forms. This sweet root acts on the adrenal glands in the body, assisting them to manage high anxiety and stress in your body. Liquorice is known as a "harmoniser", which means it is often combined with other herbs to enhance their actions in the body.

Caution: Liquorice can increase blood pressure in susceptible people, so if you have a history of high blood pressure then it is best to avoid this herb.

Rosemary

Latin: *Rosamarinus offinalis*
Herbal actions: Antidepressant, antiseptic, circulatory tonic.
Plant spirit: Rosemary brings clarity to a hazy mind, she helps you to remember the lineage of where you came from and awakens parts of you that are long forgotten.

Rosemary is a plant of the sun, giving you an idea on how it can lift the mood during times of darkness. It is stimulating to the whole body, and contains constituents that assist the liver in cleansing the system. Rosemary is easily taken as a tea, fresh, or dried. Perfect for times when you are feeling lethargic and heavy, this aromatic plant will bring the sprite back to your energy and return your zest for life.

St John's wort

Latin: *Hypericum perforatum*
Herbal actions: Alterative, astringent, nervine, antidepressant.
Plant spirit: Where there has been shock or trauma this powerful plant spirit works to restore the energy field around your body, healing the holes. Balances the solar plexus when energy is leaking out unconsciously. Brings in new levels of light and a greater connection to your soul.

A common herb for treating states of anxiety and depression, as well as a traditional remedy for neuralgia, these potent yellow flowers have a multitude of uses. As a tea or a tincture they can be very effective in lifting away any darkness of mood. These flowers bloom in the height of the summer, and they are often gathered around the summer solstice. One way to use this medicine is to make an infused oil, which when made well will turn red due to the chemical constituent hypericin. This oil can be used on the body at any time, but especially during the winter months of darkness when you feel you need some sunshine on your skin. Otherwise, both a herbal infusion or tincture are easy ways to incorporate this herb into your life.

Caution: St John's Wort is contraindicated if you are taking the contraceptive pill and anti-depressants. If you are unsure whether you can safely take this herb, then consult a medical herbalist for more information.

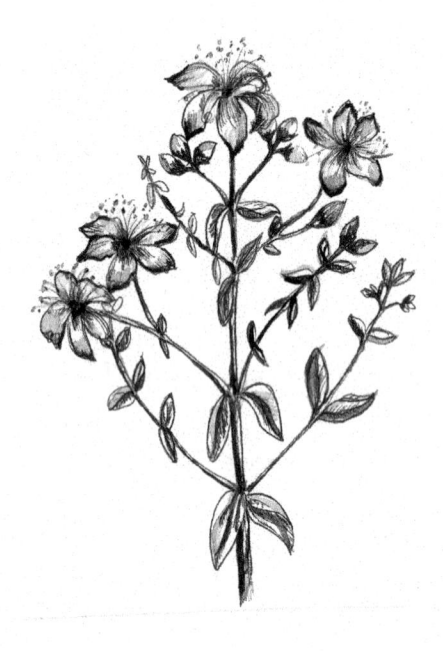

Lavender

Latin: *Lavandula officinalis*
Herbal actions: Antidepressant, sedative, carminative.
Plant spirit: Lavender awakens the spirit again with her strong presence of calm, guiding you back to a place of peace within yourself and the surrounding world.

Lavender, like many plants, evokes a variety of reactions for different people; for some it is stimulating and for others calming. If you love the smell of this beautiful flower then it is likely you will react well to the herb and it will help you to breathe deeply and ground your energy. Due to its highly aromatic scent and taste, I recommend only a small amount of this herb when mixing with other herbs so as not to create an overpowering taste. It can be taken as a tea or tincture. Lavender flowers either fresh or dried are perfect to add to any kind of bath.

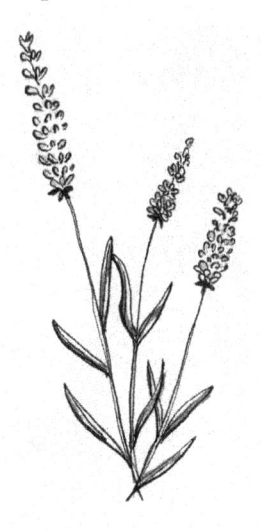

Hawthorn

Latin: *Crataegus monogyna*
Herbal actions: Cardiotonic, antioxidant, cardioprotective.
Plant spirit: The hawthorn spirit reaches deep into the heart and brings light to any darkness shrouding our lives. Her beautiful white flowers that bloom in May, symbolise all that is fertile and abundant within us.

Hawthorn is principally used as a medicine for the heart, both physically and emotionally. The leaves, flowers, and berries are safe and effective to take for any kinds of grief or trauma that you have experienced. If you are lucky enough to live near a hawthorn tree or bush, look out for the leaves and flowers as they appear in spring and have a little nibble of them. You may wish to make a fresh tea of the flowers or gather several to put into a bath later on. Even just sitting next to or beneath a hawthorn tree when feeling sad can be enough to soften any grief and offer a feeling of nourishment.

Hormones

Once the abortion is over, all the hormones that were responsible for maintaining the pregnancy will drop dramatically, which can contribute to any intense emotions or feelings that arise during this time. By understanding a few details about these changes in the body, we can become aware of how we may feel in the weeks that follow the procedure, which in turn can help those around us to give us the space we need.

One of hormones that play a key role during pregnancy is oxytocin; this is the hormone that bonds the mother to the baby even from the first moment of pregnancy. A certain state of despair that some women experience, and a sensation of feeling 'empty', may be due to the sudden drop of this hormone in the body.

Two other key hormones are oestrogen and progesterone. Oestrogen will have risen over the first few weeks of pregnancy to help the foetus develop, whilst the production of progesterone increases in order to support the uterus and the endometrium during pregnancy. As these hormones begin to rebalance it may take a while for any breast tenderness or nausea to disappear. Sometimes these symptoms can be distressing as they are a reminder of the experience you recently went through. If you feel triggered by your body, try to be kind to yourself during this time. Many do not understand what a woman is going through after an abortion, so it is up to you to realise that this is a traumatic event and to take a gentle approach to the weeks that follow to help you integrate this experience into your life. In the chapter on nutrition, I give some suggestions in terms of diet that can help rebalance hormonal fluctuations.

Symptoms that your hormones are out of balance include:

- Teariness
- Intense mood swings
- Headaches
- Insomnia
- Anxiety
- Irritability

Herbs

Agnus castus

Latin: *Vitex agnus-castus*
Herbal actions: Hormone regulator and uterine tonic.
Plant spirit: Lights the way to owning your power and creativity. Brings more confidence in your strengths and beauty, what unique gifts as a woman are you bringing into the world? Linked to the archetype of the empress.

One of the most widely used hormone balancers, agnus castus works primarily through the pituitary gland to stabilise hormonal imbalances and regulate a healthy menstrual cycle.

Agnus castus works best as a tincture; as soon as the abortion is over take 20 drops of this tincture every morning for at least 1 month. However, if you still feel unbalanced after one month, continue for another month, until your menstrual cycle has resumed and is regular. Agnus castus can be a slow working herb, so it may take several months until you start experiencing the benefits of this powerful plant.

Mugwort

Latin: *Artemisia vulgaris*
Herbal actions: Nervine, emmenagogue, diuretic.
Plant spirit: Guides you across thresholds, removes any blocks in your path, and assists the dream time and how the dream is integrated in life. Nourishes the feminine energy within and allows it to flow freely through life.

Mugwort is a relaxing and cleansing herb that helps to cleanse the body of excess blood and foetal tissue that may be left in the uterus. Combined with antiseptic properties, mugwort will help ensure that the uterus stays free from infection during and after an abortion. Another important side to this plant is how it supports the liver, which is particularly important after the pill method, as it assists the body in flushing out any antibiotics/pharmaceuticals that were used to induce an abortion.

Can be taken as a tea (bitter tasting) or tincture.
Caution: Do not take mugwort if you are still bleeding heavily as it may increase the flow. Only take it if your flow has reduced right down again.

Lady's mantle

Latin: *Alchemilla vulgaris*
Herbal actions: Astringent, antihemorrhagic, styptic.
Plant spirit: Supports and holds women as they go through challenging times. Restores self-worth and rebalances both the heart and womb space.

Lady's mantle regulates the menstrual cycle by stimulating the production of progesterone, which is an essential hormone that must be produced for regular periods. With astringent and tonic actions, lady's mantle helps tone the uterus, ensuring it returns to optimum health after the abortion.

Taken as a tea or tincture.

Herbal tea blends

Here are a couple of ideas for tea blends; the herbs mentioned below can either be taken singularly or together depending on your preference. The art of blending herbs for tea is a very personal alchemy. I encourage you to gather a few herbs that you enjoy and play around with different combinations. Soon you will discover your favourite blend.

To regain strength
- a pinch of dried sage or a couple of fresh leaves. Add a spoonful of honey to sweeten if desired.

When feeling sad
- a pinch of rose petals
- a teaspoon of dried lemon balm or a few fresh leaves.
- ½ a teaspoon of dried tulsi.

To soothe the womb
- ½ teaspoon of dried raspberry leaves or a few fresh ones.
- a small pinch of dried mugwort
- a couple of rose petals.

To bring on sleep
- a couple of fresh lime tree (*Tilia europaea*) flowers or a teaspoon of dried flowers.

- ½ teaspoon of dried chamomile.
- a pinch of dried passionflower.

For the above blends: place all of the above herbs in a mug, pour boiling water over the top, cover and leave for 10–15 minutes. Strain off the herbs and enjoy

Flower essences

Flower essences work on the energetic body, which is the energy field or aura that surrounds our physical form. They work on a very subtle level by helping the emotional state of a person to become more balanced.

The Bach flower essences are generally the most widely known; however, flower essences from all over the world are easily accessible to buy online . These subtle yet powerful plant medicines can be very effective after times of trauma, grief, and shock. By working on the subtle emotional level, this has a direct effect on our physical body, as it is often stuck or imbalanced emotions that are the root cause of illness.

Below I list a few of the Bach essences that may be helpful to take after an abortion. If you are seeking a more specific prescription then you may wish to see a flower essence practitioner, or even visit the website of flower essence makers who can guide you in choosing the right ones.[23]

- **Star of Bethlehem**—for consolation and comfort in times of grief. Brings balance and harmony.
- **Gorse**—feeling hopeless. Brings hope back into your life.
- **Sweet chestnut**—for times of anguish and despair. Brings back the light amidst any darkness.
- **Oak**—for those who endure and keep going despite hard times. Brings a realisation of limitations so that boundaries with the self can be established.
- **White chestnut**—for constant circling of thoughts and mental anguish. Brings space and peace back into one's mind.
- **Olive**—for times of exhaustion and weariness, making it challenging to continue with daily life. Encourages the need to rest and to seek support.
- **Wild rose**—a feeling of resignation coupled with loss of interest for life. Brings vitality.

- **Honeysuckle**—to help move past the pain of the past, and return to the peaceful present.
- **Cerato**—to restore sense of confidence, and release yourself from the judgement of others. You know what is best for yourself.

Self care

Womb massage

What is Womb Massage?
It is a series of gentle strokes that we can perform on our lower abdomen to help nurture our connection with this part of our body and to increase blood flow, bringing healing energy to our wombs.

How to Do a Womb Massage?
The illustrations below demonstrate how to do a womb massage. I recommend that you use an oil, as this will cause less friction on the skin. If you already have a favourite body oil then this will be perfect, if not then some simple almond or olive oil would be absolutely fine. If you fancy making an infused oil, then I would recommend chamomile, rose or calendula as herbs that you could use singularly or blended together as a healing oil for your womb.

When to do a Womb Massage?
The answer is whenever you feel ready to connect with that part of your body again. Depending on your own abortion journey, this could be the day after or months later. There is no rush, healing takes all the time it needs.

As this is a very gentle massage it can be done at any time. However, whilst you are bleeding you may feel very sensitive; if so, then it is a good idea to wait until the bleeding has ended before you begin a massage. Yet, there is nothing stopping you from simply lying down and connecting with your womb space at any point by simply by laying your hands over this area.

Why do a Womb Massage?
After an abortion it is common for women to feel disconnected from their womb space, this could be due to feelings of shame, grief, or trauma.

By engaging in this simple practice you can begin to heal the relationship with your womb, bringing much needed healing to this part of your body. If a massage feels like too much, then even just a simple daily commitment of placing your hands over your womb can be enough to restore connection and bring a sense of grounded peace to your being.

1. Lie down somewhere comfortable and warm. Place a cushion or blanket underneath your knees to support your lower back.
2. Place your hands over your womb, a couple of inches below your belly button. Spend a few moments tuning into this space in your body. How does it feel? Can you feel any heat radiating through the skin? Simply feel the rise and fall of your breath on your belly.
3. Is there an intention that you wish to make before you begin? It could be to connect with your womb, to bring healing energy, or to give thanks to this space. Allow whatever comes to mind and choose to hold this intention throughout the massage.
4. Now put a small amount of oil on your belly, and beginning at your womb space, start to move your hands clockwise around your belly button. Using only gentle pressure as you continue to circulate the belly.
5. As you massage your hands in slow circles, you may notice some tender spots where less pressure is needed, or spots where you are called to stay in that one place. Allow your hands to travel to where they are drawn to.
6. Allow 10–20 minutes of time to do this massage. To begin with this may seem a long time, though the more often you practice it, the longer you may wish to hold this connection with your womb space.
7. Once you have finished the massage, hold your hands over your womb and take a couple of big belly breaths. Notice how you are feeling. Finally, gently emerge from this space and give yourself thanks for spending these moments connecting to your body.

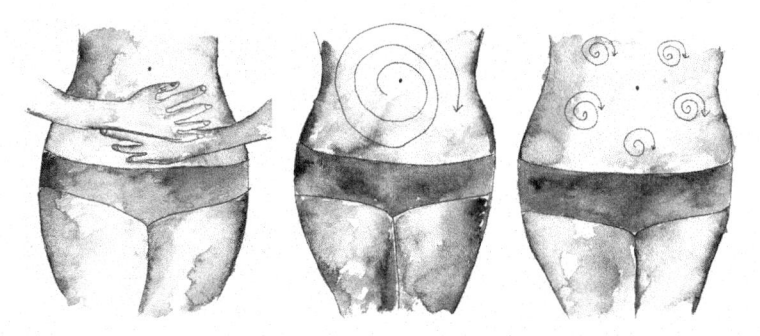

Fig. 1. Massage 1.   Fig. 2. Massage 2.   Fig. 3. Massage 3.

CHAPTER 4

Long term after an abortion

"Acceptance is simply the strength to face, experience and integrate your losses".[24]

The journey to being truly at peace with your abortion can be a long and spiralling one. There is no timeline for when you must feel "over it"; some women feel ready to move on after a few months, for others it could be years. As I mentioned earlier when talking about how our society regards death, as well as the taboo that still surrounds abortion, there can be a tendency to feel like we have to close the door on our experience quickly, that it may seem silly to still have a cry about it three years later, but it is not. Our emotions are signals telling us that something wants to be released from within. They are a healthy sign that we have the capacity to feel deeply about life, they are our truth and when listened to, can open us up to trusting our inner feelings and moving into a deeper relationship with ourselves.

As the years pass after the abortion, the grief may lessen as you come to terms with the experience. However, as with all major life experiences, traumatic memories and grief can resurface at any given moment. Each time a memory returns, we have the choice of how we tend to this memory. Do we greet it with love and kindness, or does pain and hurt emerge from these thoughts? If you feel enveloped by the latter, then it can be helpful to hold your hands over your womb (lower belly), take a few deep breaths and gently sit with these feelings.

You may wish to contemplate these questions:

Do you feel like you need support to work through your abortion journey?

Is there anyone around you who you can speak to when you feel overwhelmed by your feelings?

> "We must turn towards our experience and touch it with the softest hands possible".[25]

There is a difference between still being traumatised by an abortion that happened many years ago and simply feeling sadness resurface from time to time. If you have experienced persistent symptoms of depression following your abortion, such as a low mood, lack of enjoyment in previously rewarding activities, sleep or eating disturbances, then it may be wise to seek professional help with someone who can support you in slowly coming to terms with what happened.

Ultimately this experience has become part of you and the rich tapestry of your life. I am not asking you to embrace it, if that is not how you feel, but rather encouraging you to give space to the feelings, sensations, and emotions that arise in you when memories of the abortion resurface. By creating this space, you are honouring what was hidden within you and allowing it to gently rise to the surface. The emergence of these challenging feelings may cause you to instinctively react to suppress them.

However, by allowing that feeling of guilt or shame, for example, to come into your awareness, you are on the path to releasing these feelings. This may seem counterproductive, yet despite any understandable fear of becoming engulfed by these sensations, the reverse is what occurs. Although this transformation may not be instant, through a commitment to work through these feelings of the past, you are taking steps in the right direction towards looking at your abortion with acceptance and peace.

There are an infinite number of ways that an abortion may have affected you, ways that you may never have imagined and often go unspoken. From anger, guilt, and shame, to issues surrounding intimacy, and fears of infertility or having to go through it again, to mention but a few. There is no right way to feel; some women may even feel no grief at all from their experience. Although this is a minority, it demonstrates how we each travel through this time in a way that is unique to ourselves.

There is no one formula to healing from an abortion, this is a slow and steady journey that when approached gently and with courage will hopefully lead you to a place of peace. This can take an immense amount of inner strength and affirmation that you are worthy of healing. That is the first step; realising that amidst any shame, guilt, or regret, you are worthy of acknowledging these emotions as real, and in doing so you sow a seed of desire to bring healing to these hidden places within you.

> "While something may come to an ending on the surface of time, its presence, meaning and effect continue to be held and integrated in the eternal".[26]

Sharing your experience

> "If we can share our story with someone who responds with empathy and understanding, shame can't survive".[27]

Abortion is a controversial and contested subject within many modern cultures, and a polarised debate exists within some political and religious contexts. This controversy is not conducive to an environment where women feel safe to tell their abortion story, hence the secrecy that surrounds this topic. It can be therapeutic to share your experience, or if you would rather keep it close to your chest then I hope that there are some caring listening ears around you who one day may hear what you have to say without judgement.

Since the beginning of time, women have been gathering in circle, to share their stories and support each other through the trials and tribulations of life. It can often take one brave friend in a group to share their experience of abortion before other women around them feel comfortable to share theirs. If you have never ventured into the soothing space of a women's circle, but are intrigued to explore this possibility then check out "Red Tents". They are circles of women who gather together usually around the new or full moon to simply sit together, chat, sing, and dance. The circle is made up of mostly strangers, and one of their foundational principles is confidentiality. These safe women-held spaces can become a lifeline amidst difficult experiences.

If you feel unsure about being in a circle with strangers, you could send a message to the facilitator of the space and let her know your fears about coming. She will hopefully put your mind at ease and warmly welcome you to the space.

> "This was the most personal of journeys, and I have grieved it and found meaning and empowerment in myriad ways through it. And the support of sisterhood, of women who have known this and haven't known this has been the biggest balm of non-judgemental support".
>
> —C.G.

My hope is that one day abortion may be truly accepted without judgement the world over; giving women the freedom to speak up about their experience, so that no woman has to suffer in silence. Up until that moment, we as women must be responsible for supporting other women through these difficult times. Showing younger generations how we can come together and hold space for those who are suffering, by acknowledging their pain as real and offering our love and compassion towards our sisters.

How long ago?

Depending on how many months or years ago that you had an abortion, you may be experiencing a wide range of post-abortion physical and emotions symptoms.

Months—If the experience was only recent, you may still be bleeding as your hormones work hard to rebalance your body again. If you are lucky then your period will have returned, bringing with it a certain rhythmic normality into your life (unless you are on contraception).

The experience could still feel raw, and you would rather not go there. Begin by taking small and gentle steps within your capacity, this could be having more baths than usual or sleeping in to allow your body to rest and recover. Abortion after-care does not have to be extensive and complicated; ultimately it is about recognising that you are allowed to listen to the needs of your body during this challenging time.

Often the time when the baby was due is a significant moment for many women in their healing process. If you have the date lodged in your mind, then why not choose to honour that day in a small way. Maybe there is a strong desire to become pregnant again against all logic and rational thinking. This natural feeling is the body trying to replace what was lost, and could be partly why it is incredibly easy to become pregnant very soon after an abortion. Maybe there are psychological effects, such as trauma around sex and intimacy, fears about becoming pregnant again, or shame about the decision that you made.

Accepting whatever is coming up for you in these months, and reaching out for support when you need it, will help you travel through this time with greater ease and ultimately aid your long-term healing.

Years—Your abortion was years ago, yet the memories surrounding the experience are still easily accessible. There are many factors that could have played a role in determining how you feel about the experience all these years later; from what your life looked like at the time of the abortion to the presence or lack of support network around you.

When speaking to women who had an abortion over a decade ago, I found that the experience was still etched in their memory. Often when one goes through this challenging time during our younger years, we felt like we had no resources that we could call on to help us through, so the experience was dismissed and life carried on. Yet it is only in the years later that opportunities arise for us to journey back to that time and allow any feelings or emotions to surface as we feel strong enough to honour the loss that was.

In the years following an abortion, there can be certain moments that trigger a cascade of emotions, such as becoming pregnant again along with the choice of how you wish to go on and supporting friends or family through pregnancies and baby loss. Later on in life, as the shift towards menopause begins to take place, there is often a time where women review and reflect upon their whole reproductive history. This opens up a new space for any buried grief or strong emotions to emerge from within and through feeling them they are transformed. In the journey of life, it is never too late or the wrong time to grieve; when we find the support and space that we need, even if that is twenty years later, this opens a space inside of us to let go of anything we have been holding onto during all those years. Life is always giving us opportunities to heal our pain, all we need to do is trust that all we need is revealed to us and we are wonderful as we are. In this mind-set, we are open to any moments that act as catalysts for great transformation to occur, and ultimately to feel a greater inner peace.

Grief

> "We can also share our grief with a tree or a riverbank, in writing or in clay. We can dance our grief or express it through music".[28]

The psychotherapist and holder of ritual spaces, Francis Weller, talks about having "faith in grief"; how grief is a journey that we all are taken on at various moments in our lives, and by acknowledging it we are opening the door to a greater capacity to love. Grief shows us that we truly loved something or someone, and we are now mourning that loss. It is a sign that we opened our hearts to feel the depth of that wondrous and ever powerful emotion, love.

When we begin to see that grief is showing us our enormous capacity to love, then the perspective shifts and we can begin to truly honour the process of grieving. This can be tough, especially in a society that does not offer the ancient ways of moving through grief with ritual and ceremony.

There may be many different aspects of grief present, each one connecting to a different element of going through an abortion. Some women may resonate with one, others with all of them or none. Different sides can present themselves at various times over the following months and years after an abortion, it can be a slow unfolding of many layers. There is no right way to feel, only to feel what is true for you.

> "I had a counselling session a few months later, when I was still swimming in guilt and regret. I was guided through the 'Gestalt' practice of using different chairs to dialogue with the being who would have been my baby. I offered my heartfelt apologies and something of what I felt. When I swapped to sit in the seat that represented the baby it said very clearly to me 'It is what it is' and I felt no anger or ill will from the baby towards me".
>
> — C.G

The many sides of grief

For some, intense feelings are entwined with the trauma of the experience. Were you supported in your decision? Were you alone? Or with a partner or friend? Were the doctors/nurses supportive?

For other women the grief is linked to the decision they made; as they process their experience, they may find themselves filled with guilt, regret, and shame. In working through these feelings, take your time to source the root of them. This is complex, as the root could come from societal, religious, or family values. If you feel overwhelmed by the weight of your decision, then it is always best to seek professional support and guidance.

A broader perspective on the forms of grief is in thinking about why women choose to have an abortion. This again is complex and each woman will have one or several reasons for her choice. However, for some, the grief is there long before the abortion. Grief for the lack of tribe and community within society, a safe protected space where women knew they would be supported with bringing new life in the world. Or grief for the state of the planet; where the world seems and uninhabitable and a hostile place to bring up children. Experiencing these wider forms of grief may cause much sorrow. Yet, we all hold the power to change the world and from these dark places; new seeds are gestating to be born, so that we can create a world that feels solid, safe, and peaceful to welcome new life.

All these forms of grief can merge into each other, manifesting as an inner block that feels insurmountable. By choosing to open the doorway to your experience and by being present in a non-judgemental space with yourself, you take the first step to mending the fractured parts of your inner being, and calling them back to your heart.

We all grieve in different ways; whilst some require solitude, others seek community. As you move through your own process, see if you can feel what it is that you need. This could be taking a day away from work to go on a long walk, or calling your friends together to drink tea and chat. Even in the most hopeless of times, sometimes the tiniest gesture towards yourself can make the world of difference.

Ways to cope with grief

Here are a few suggestions of what to do when you suddenly feel knocked down by a wave of grief or strong emotions. These feelings could come out of nowhere or be triggered by any arising memories of your experience.

- Make a cup of tea with any of the soothing herbs that I mention in Chapter 2 and 3. Spend a quiet moment with your cup of tea, drinking in the healing powers of the herbs and breathing deeply as you move through the intensity of the moment.
- Call a trusted friend or family member that can offer non-judgemental support. Talk to them about how you are feeling. It can be daunting to reach out to talk about an experience that many supress and dismiss until many years later. This may provoke feelings of vulnerability, as you open yourself up to someone else. Know that in being vulnerable you are also being immensely brave, by consciously choosing to witness and express the depths of your feelings.
- Being in nature, the ultimate seat of life and loss, can help if feelings are overwhelming. Paying close attention to all the ways in which life comes and goes. Immerse yourself in the sea or a river, allow your contact with the earth to support and ground you, or just go for a walk in the sunshine/pouring rain—this can ease or shift pain.
- Curl up and have a nap; giving yourself permission to rest is a radical act in today's busy world.
- Grief is often felt in the body as much as the mind. Find ways to move or engage with your body, through activities such as meditation, chi-gung, or yoga. This may help your feelings loosen and ebb.
- Create a physical space, like a shrine or alter, that honours your experience as a woman. You can include pictures or symbols of women you admire, or energies you find supportive, and spend time there when feelings of grief or gratitude are strong. It could be as simple as a special candle that sits on your kitchen table that you light when feelings about your abortion are strong, creating a focus for your feelings.
- If you feel stuck in your grief, where nothing you do makes you feel better, then reach out for some professional support to guide you.

> "Despite being in constant communication with the soul who passed through my body, I was in a place of deep grief and craved connection with my partner at the time. In the months that followed, although the grief lessened, it would have the power to throw me back into its grip. I learnt to go with these moments, allowing them to unfold and seek support from those around me".
>
> —I.H

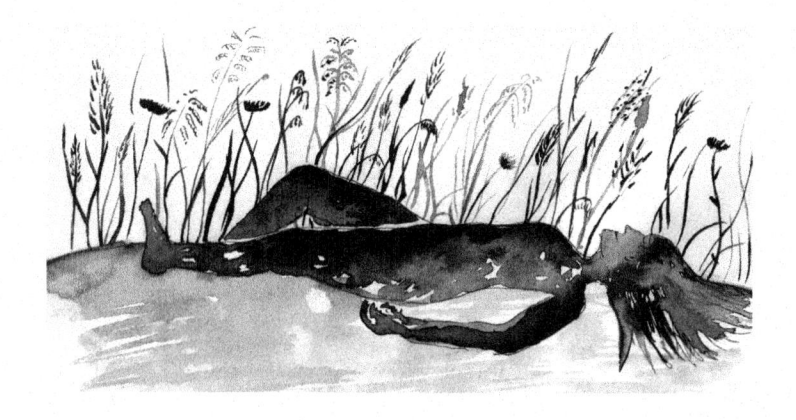

The act of blessing

Blessing is a lost art within our language and daily life. Aside from the role that blessing plays in religion, we no longer know how to involve this gentle act into our lives. The etymology of the word from Old English is "to consecrate by a religious rite, make holy, give thanks".[29] To make holy can also mean to make *sacred*. When we bless something, we are choosing to elevate it to beyond the ordinary. Therefore, giving thanks for all that we are grateful for in our lives.

A blessing is a form of healing using the gift of words. We may wish to bless our bodies, our wombs, our friends or our life. When we speak a blessing this opens the doors for healing to happen in a way that is not religious, just simply a way to convey love and gratitude towards something.

> "The word *blessing* evokes a sense of warmth and protections, it suggests that no life is alone or unreachable".[30]

In the time following an abortion, a blessing can be done towards any aspect of the experience; such as the baby loss, your womb, or your heart. If you establish this as a regular practice, it can become a useful tool to use whenever you feel challenging emotions surface in the months and years after. As Tami Lynn Kent says, "Blessings work on the deeper layers to heal our spiritual fractures: these places we have lost touch with spirit. Blessings are a salve that we can use to restore our inherent wholeness".[31]

You can create your own blessing by writing down the words that feel appropriate to you, or simply say aloud what you choose to bless. Here is a womb blessing you may choose to use.

A Blessing for a womb after an abortion

Sacred container of life,
I ask for your forgiveness.
One moment you held a tiny one within your walls,
Then it was gone.
I am sorry for your pain,
I too am hurting,
Let us gently heal together.
May I honour your gifts of renewal,
By blessing the
Ever-cyclical, creative centre of
My universe that you are
are.
Blessed Be.

Herbal healing

The broad spectrum of time after an abortion means that there is no specific remedy for the body. In Chapter 3 I cover a whole range of possible symptoms that could easily apply to the months after an abortion. Therefore, if you are only a month or two post-abortion and feel like your body is still imbalanced, then I would recommend that you read through the different herbs that I mention throughout the book, to find out which ones may be help you to rebalance your body.

The long-term effects of an abortion are likely to be more psychological than physical; therefore, the herbs that I recommend are ones for the *nervous system* and *grief*. The role of herbs for this time involves acts of self-care, such as baths, massage oils, vagina steams, and balms.

The menstrual cycle and the moon

The word menstrual originates from the word Moon—worth a ponder into the mysteries of being a woman.

An abortion can often be a wake-up call to one's own fertility, especially if you have never had a child before. We all know in varying degrees of detail that around ovulation is when we can get pregnant; however, this very fertile window can seem like a mythical moment until suddenly we find ourselves pregnant. Although some women may become pregnant in the months following one, for most the aim is to not become pregnant involuntarily again. By learning more about the natural cycle of your womb each month, you can become more empowered in your body and help to prevent another unwanted pregnancy.

If you feel that since your experience you would like to learn more about the menstrual cycle and the different phases that each woman moves through each month then be prepared for a fascinating journey into the essence of being a woman.

Over the last ten years, there has been a surge in menstrual awareness, a new concept for the generation of our mothers and grandmothers who grew up in a time when "period" was a dirty word that you never spoke of. However, this movement to de-stigmatise menstruation is powerful and ever-increasing in momentum, as women begin to wake-up to the enormous creative power that is held within their wombs.

What are the benefits to understanding your menstrual cycle?

- Knowing the length of your cycle, so you can better predict when your period will arrive.
- Becoming aware of the days you feel like hiding from the world, and the other days that you feel like changing the world.
- Knowing when you are fertile, useful if you are practicing natural contraception and/or wish to become or avoid getting pregnant.
- Creating a more harmonious relationship with partners. As you begin to notice monthly patterns in moods and sensations, you may choose to share your findings with them. This can help in your partner understanding why some days you crave closeness and intimacy and on other days you seek the opposite.
- Becoming empowered in your body's own inherent rhythms, which have a direct positive impact on how you view and accept your body in all her forms.

Life is a spiral

Learning about your cycle is an empowering and sometimes life-changing journey. As you tap into the different phases and "seasons" within each month, a greater acceptance of yourself as an ever-changing, cyclical, and spiralling woman occurs. Most of us are born into a linear male dominated society, where the focus is on non-stop achieving and doing. This leaves little space for the female part of ourselves that requires time to create, to be and live in our own cyclical way. As women, we must forge our own path within this imbalanced state of the world; by living our truth, and not falling for the pitfalls of the patriarchy.

Within our own individual life experiences, we will have lived through many twists and turns, joys and set-backs that life offers, there is no straight path. Women have their own radar of how to live life that is true to their nature, this is called their menstrual cycle. Although the external world may tell us that we must be constantly striving and expressing all our energy, our bodies can't maintain such an intense existence forever. This is why we become much more susceptible to illness when we are run down and exhausted, rest is essential to our wellbeing, especially as women.

In seeking a true example of how to live in a cyclical way, we can turn to nature, who effortlessly transitions from one season to another. Nature exemplifies how we are constantly moving through cycles of birth and death, both on the earth we live in and within our female bodies.

In winter when the light is low, the trees are stripped bare, and the air is cold, our bodies instinctively seek more rest and nourishment. This time of hibernation is for replenishing and restoring ourselves so that when spring arrives, we are full of energy and creativity to flourish back into the world again. As the weather heats up and summer emerges, the bounty of nature is shown through the fields of flowers and beauty. This is nature at her fullest. Slowly, as late summer arrives with the seed heads and drying of stems showing the signs of autumn, the circle turns again with the light decreasing and a shedding of the old to return again into the dark space of winter.

This way of living is deeply feminine, and one that many of us have lost touch with. Yet the joy of being a woman is that we have our menstrual cycles as a tool to help us live in a way that is ancient, healing, and harmonious with the natural world.

The seasons of the womb

Each month our womb journeys through four different phases, according to what is both physically and energetically happening in the body. This way of connecting our womb's cycle with that of the earth is ancient; however, in recent times there are several inspiring teachers who speak wisely of these rhythms and have been instrumental in returning this wisdom to women. One is Alexandra Pope and the other is Jewels Wingfield. In the Resources section, I have included many fantastic resources and books for those who wish to delve deeper into this fascinating topic.

Winter—Menstruation. Our bleeding days are when our focus goes within; maybe our dreams become lucid and more potent. There is less energy to complete projects and start new ones. It is the time to rest.

Spring—The follicular phase. The ovaries are maturing the egg ready for secretion. Our energy is returning as we have stopped bleeding and our wombs are feeling light again. With the rise in hormones oestrogen and testosterone, libido returns as we welcome a fresh and inquisitive outlook on the world.

Summer—Ovulation. The height of our cycle, when the egg has now been released from the ovaries into the fallopian tube. We may feel intense energy in our bodies, a sense that we must create. This is an easy time to burnout with all this energy to play with.

Autumn—The luteal phase. If not fertilised, the egg breaks down and the lining of the womb prepares to be released as blood during the next period. This is a time of transition, when symptoms of PMS may arise. This is a time to take particularly good care of yourself, including lots of sleep and recognising the need to be alone.

How to track your menstrual cycle

1. Using a calendar.
   Noting down on a calendar which day you start your period each month is a great start to tracking your cycle. Over a few months this will show you if you have a regular (within 2/3 days) or irregular cycle. You may also begin to notice other elements to your cycle, such as bleeding near the new or full moon.

   As well as writing down any physical changes, begin to notice the emotional shifts that happen throughout the month. This will bring another aspect of awareness to your monthly rhythms, as you discover the correlation between your moods and where you are in your cycle.

2. Basal body temperature.
The basal body temperature, or BBT, is the temperature of your body taken around the same time every morning before you get out of bed. This daily temperature is one of the most accurate ways to see where you are in your cycle, as directly after ovulation your BBT will rise several decimal points. This is caused by the hormone progesterone, which has a heating effect on the body after it is produced following ovulation. Generally, for the rest of the cycle your BBT will stay higher than the first half. Another shift in the BBT will occur just before your period, maybe on the day or a day or two before, the temperature will drop indicating its arrival. Keeping track of your BBT is crucial if you are keen to really get to know your own cycle, there are many forms of charts that are easily downloadable. This way requires discipline, but is well worth it for the knowledge that will be gained from using it.

3. Cervical mucus.
Cervical mucus (CM) changes dramatically throughout your cycle as you may have noticed. From feeling like it is pouring out your body, to being a bit sticky and then to none at all, these are all indicators of your fertility.

Often just after your period your cervical mucus will be a bit sticky or non-existent, this is generally a sign that you are not fertile, A sign that you are approaching ovulation is when your cervical mucus becomes very clear and runny, almost like egg-whites. This is your body providing the perfect liquid that will help the sperm travel up and reach the egg. Once ovulation is over, then the cervical mucus is likely to decrease and become thicker in consistency. After several months of paying attention to your CM, you will begin to become much more aware of how it changes throughout the month and how those changes correlate with all the other aspects of your menstrual cycle.

4. Position of your cervix.
If you were to put your finger into your vagina and reach up as high as you could go, you may be able to reach your cervix. For most of

your cycle it will feel hard, however during the phase of ovulation it will feel soft and squishy.

During, just before and after your period the cervix is lower down in your vagina, this is when you may be able to feel it. During ovulation, it rises higher up so that it shortens the distance for any possible sperm to travel before meeting an egg.

Tracking your cycle with an app

There are various apps, such as Clue, Flo and Ovio amongst others, that can be a fantastic way in to period tracking. As useful as they are, your own intuition will guide you far more reliably than an app. So if you choose to use an app, then stay mindful of what you are feeling both physically and emotionally throughout the month and see if that corresponds with the algorithms created. There is something very empowering about dedicating a journal to what is going on inside your body; it becomes a creative process that can nourish every aspect of your life.

A final word on periods

Once you begin noticing all the changes that occur to you throughout the month, you will start to feel the changes of your inner season more clearly. This journey of learning about our bodies takes time and many months of careful observation and discipline. Yet with discipline comes freedom, and this freedom is found through a deep and connected relationship with your body, allowing you to intimately harmonise with the ebbs and flows of your cycle and, consequently, all of life.

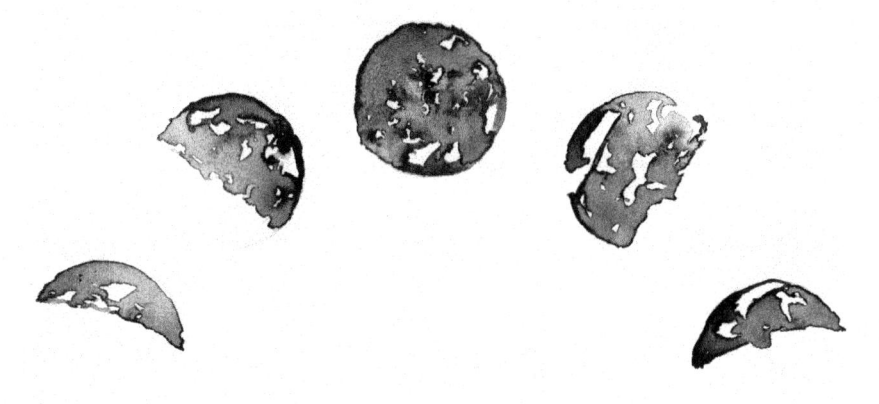

The moon

The moon, who represents all things feminine and unconscious, has been a guide to women's bodies since the beginning of time. She who cycles through the night, waxing and waning in her cyclical way can become a magical ally to all who wish to get to know her. As a ruler of the waters, the moon affects us all regardless of gender. We only need to start to notice the behaviour of those around us on a full moon compared to a new moon to realise the impact she has on us.

Back in the day when our bodies were not disrupted by artificial lights and we lived closer to the rhythms of the earth, it was thought that women would bleed together on the new moon and ovulate during the full moon. Although many women's cycles are no longer in sync with the moon, there are many ways to attune to the lunar cycle and consequently feel more connected to her ancient and powerful energies.

If after the abortion you are planning on beginning a form of contraception that will result in your period disappearing, however you wish to stay connected to the ebb and flow of your cycle, then this is where the moon comes in. As with the seasons of the menstrual cycle there is also a corresponding moon phase to tune into. Below is a simple diagram of how it is possible to connect with the greater rhythms of nature despite not having a monthly period.

Ways to connect to the moon

- On a full moon night head outside and bathe in the moon rays.
- Take a bath on the full moon to connect to the waters, asking the full moon to cleanse you of all you wish to let go of.
- Note down the changes that you feel between a new moon and a full moon.
- On a new moon, spend a few moments outside feeling the darkness envelop you. This can also be done in your room with all the lights off.
- How do your dreams change throughout the month?

Natural contraception — cycle awareness method

The introduction I give into tracking your cycle is not detailed enough to guide you through practicing natural contraception, it is only to give a brief introduction into this way of understanding your body. If you are interested in moving away from other forms of contraception and just using your body, then it is very important that you already have a strong connection with the phases of your cycle before you go full time no other protection. At the back of this book there is a list of fantastic books and tools which will help guide you along the journey to practicing natural contraception, often called the "Fertility Awareness Method".

CHAPTER 5

Rituals

"We are creatures of ritual"[32]
All over the world, rituals are incorporated into the daily lives of many cultures and indigenous peoples. From honouring the morning sun on the eastern horizon to making offerings to a special deity; rituals can take a multitude of forms, yet they all share a similar thread of consciously choosing to weave the sacred into life. Within these ancient cultures, ritual is woven throughout the lives of the people, who live with an intimate knowledge of the earth's rhythms and cycles.

One reason that we may crave ritual in the West is because of our lack of connection with each other, the land, and our ancestors. We are seeking a meaningful connection with life and something larger than us. The need for ritual can be a longing that comes from deep within our bones, maybe in the form of a dream or just a feeling that nudges us to mark the sacredness of a moment. Rituals are an alchemy of intention, conscious action, and sacred space, this combination creates a doorway of transformation from one state of being to another, allowing shifts to occur in both our inner and outer worlds.

As women, ritual runs deep through our blood, although we have mostly forgotten the significance of this word. As we begin working with ritual again, this can become an act of reclaiming the word and remembering both our ability and right to create sacred space in our lives. For some the word can bring up strictly religious connotations or old history lessons of bloody rituals that may have occurred in various traditions; however, this word goes back to the beginning of time long before any patriarchal structures attempted to conform the ancient ways.

Rituals make your actions sacred and special, they ask you to focus on every element, by creating an intention that is connected with what you wish to transform. There are many layers to the word; for some, ritual brings to mind their family traditions when gathering together during festive moments. In this case, the ritual is a time for community and reminds them of the seasons of life. For others, ritual suggests moments of communing with spirit in a sacred space. Here the focus is more specific, where the intention is to open up to the other world. We all have our own way of interpreting the word depending on our culture and traditions; ultimately when we chose to weave ritual into our lives, we are stepping outside of the normal timeframe of life and stepping into a space where anything is possible.

Ritual and abortion

Each woman is on her own journey of healing after an abortion. For some, the central feeling may be relief and joy, whilst for others they are deep in the grief and trauma of the experience. Regardless of how you may be feeling, you have been through a significant loss and ritual can be a useful tool to bring balance back into your life and body. Often, after an abortion we can feel disconnected and cut off from our womb, as feelings of guilt and shame emerge from within. If left unresolved, this disconnection from this part of your body can remain with you for many years, having a negative impact on aspects of your life that are linked with your womb, such as your menstrual cycle, having sex, or even getting pregnant again. If you resonate with this feeling of disconnect, and wish to nourish this part of your body, begin to explore some of these rituals and self-care practices that will ever so gently encourage a nourishing bond to form between you and your womb.

Sometimes, the emotional state that many women find themselves in after an abortion can be the reason for seeking ritual to honour their experiences. When tough emotions arise there may be the feeling of wanting them to just go away, and although ritual can revolve around the desire to transform one state of feeling to another, the change is not necessarily about getting those feelings to disappear, as this can take time. It is more about consciously creating space within to accept those feelings, which ultimately leads towards transformation.

For me, when we decide to mark a loss through ritual, however big or small, we are not only honouring ourselves and our experience, but we are also honouring our mothers, grandmothers, great grandmothers and beyond who had and maybe lost babies. We are honouring our ancestors who lived in harmony with the dance of life and death, and inviting this ancient way of being back into our lives again.

Why create a ritual after an abortion?

Living in a world where abortion is often illegal or strongly frowned upon can create a feeling of unworthiness within us. Such an environment may cause us to wonder, how can choosing to have an abortion be worthy of ritual? are we allowed to honour something that is deemed a taboo? These thoughts only encourage us to quickly continue with our busy lives as before, despite a grey shadow hanging over us. I wish to address a desire that some women may feel in the time following an abortion, the desire to acknowledge the experience, through creating a sacred space that honours the loss and nourishes your soul.

Ritual offers a space to listen to our hearts and wombs, witness them fully, and create a way to release any pain or grief. Something as simple as lighting a candle or taking some body oil and gently massaging your womb can begin to heal a disconnect that may have occurred as a result of the abortion. As Jackie Singer, author of *Birthrites*, mentions, "At times of grief, ritual offers a container that is deep and strong enough to hold intense emotions".[33]

Ritual asks us to honestly sit with ourselves and our actions; this is a courageous move and one that can bring up some heavy emotions. Although many of the rituals I have included are ones that can be done alone, many are an opportunity to involve someone you love and trust into this moment to share the transformation together.

Passing through a threshold

A threshold is a space between what was and what is to come. We stand in this liminal space during various moments of life; they signify a change is coming. The two thresholds that we all travel through are birth and death, and those whom have female bodies will know that throughout our lives, our wombs signify moments of change in the form of either beginning our menstrual years or ending them. These moments are life changing, yet in today's world we have forgotten how to truly honour these times. As the poet John Donohue says, "When we stand before crucial thresholds in our lives, we have no rituals to protect, encourage and guide us as we cross over into the unknown".[34]

A threshold represents a transition into the unknown. There is no knowing how we will feel when we wake up the day after our abortion, yet through the experience we are somehow changed. We entered the liminal space between life and death so briefly, yet with a marked moment that remains in our memories.

> "I woke up the day after my abortion a different woman, I had crossed a new threshold which involved death, I felt grateful to be alive and to be given the gift of freedom. The experience had felt like an initiation that I had never planned to take, one that continues to unfold all these years later and provides me with deep compassion for every other woman who experienced this too."
>
> —I.H.

Ritual is a tool we can use to help us through this threshold of change and transition. By creating an intention and holding a sacred space, profound shifts can be made, allowing a greater sense of peace and wellbeing to flow into one's life. Abortion is a time of transition for both you, your body and the little being growing inside in your womb. Through creating a ritual or being part of one, this simple act can bring a greater sense of harmony with what happened and assist in the integration of this change in your life during the months and years after. Every woman is on her own journey, for some they may be able to engage in a ritual straight away or for others the idea of creating a ritual so soon may be too much, and the right time comes later on. Trust your own judgement and feelings towards the timing of everything.

Here is a beautiful account from a friend who created her own ritual to honour the loss of her abortion, and how she arrived to a place of acceptance.

> "I felt strongly that it was a girl and I sat dazed in the toilet. I wrapped it up in loo roll and a blue cloth and encouraged my friend to leave without telling him what had happened. I slept that

night with the wrapped bundle next to my heart. I felt that the fact that it took 4 days to pass reflected my uncertainty and my body's wish to hang on to it. I didn't do this lightly.

The next day I buried it in the garden. It was beautiful and lonely and I didn't think I'd done it right. I rang my best friend who was a trainee teacher and told her what had happened. She went back into the school and the head teacher saw her in the corridor looking like she'd seen a ghost. She called her into her office and asked what had happened. She said, 'My best friend has just had a very traumatic miscarriage' and the head teacher said 'Was it on purpose?' She'd guessed and said to my friend 'You must go to her at once, of course you must, take the rest of the week off.' I was never more grateful to a human I have never met.

Once my friend arrived we settled and wept together, and played 'Down to the river to pray' on repeat as we reburied the tiny box together, deeper and more securely and with more ceremony. I wore a necklace all the time then, and I put that in the box as well. It felt like a part of me would always be with this being.

Like so many women I could have wrapped myself in a blanket of grief and regret and shame and berated myself. There was some of that but some things really helped.

I slept with the blue cloth scrunched up for more than a year, close to my heart. A friend came to stay at one point and unfurled it and wrapped me in it—that gave it space. There came a point two years later when I burned it and released some of the grief.

At the dump, not long after, I randomly found two wooden carvings on the edge of a bin, in the shape of my necklace but open at the top. Over time, I painted them green, and one sits where the being that would have been my baby is buried, and one sits on my alter.

I went on a meditation retreat in the January, and my heart, where the cloth was held was so painful. I forgave myself that week, and never since have I berated the person I was then for the decision I made then. I was leading a pretty unconscious, unhappy life at the time, and this being came into my life for a short time to wake me up, to remind me that this life is a miracle and that things have consequences, and now I share any merit that I make with the being that would have been my baby."

—C.G.

Creating our own rituals

Many of us have lost our indigenous roots and may be wondering, how can we authentically connect with ritual when the lineage of our ancient teachings are lost? The solution lies in our own inherent wisdom and creativity. With a helping hand to guide us and show us the way, we can begin to create authentic and embodied rituals for significant moments in our lives.

Often people turn to indigenous cultures for inspiration on how to acknowledge a loss, using their rituals as examples. However, often we are not aware of the true context of those rituals or why and when to apply them. This is a delicate subject as often we are not born into or part of those ancient cultures despite maybe feeling a longing to be.

We may be inspired by rituals that are rooted in other cultures, yet they are not ours to copy and claim as our own. Instead, look for the thread that joins all rituals across the world together. This thread is of honouring, blessing, and giving thanks. When we consider those words as a root to our own rituals, it gives us a base to work from. What do we want to give thanks for? To honour or transform?

Take smudging for example, a popular way of cleansing a space or person, using the smoke of white sage (*Salvia apiana*). This ritual comes from the Native Americans, yet across the world many of us reach for white sage when we wish to cleanse away the old with this sacred smoke. However, questions have been raised about whether the industry of growing this particular sage is sustainable. It is a healthy question to ask, and one that has caused a shift in looking for ways to continue cleansing spaces with plants. When looking into the history of the herbs that the Celts and Druids used for smoke cleansing, the list is long and full of our native plants, such as rosemary, sage, and mugwort. These native plants are as potent as the white sage and although their energy is different and they have their own unique attributes, they were all used for good reason by the ancestors of this land.

We each have our own heritage rich in traditions and rituals, as we delve deeper into these stories and begin to learn which plants our ancestors used for one thing or another, we begin to heal the void of lost knowledge. If you are aware of your ancestral heritage then you may choose to do some research into the plants your ancestors used; this could involve going to a botanical garden to see the plants in the flesh, or ordering them from a reputable supplier. The greater your relationship is with the plants you use in ritual, the stronger the ritual is. However, if to craft a ritual with plants doesn't require knowledge of ancestral usage of those plants, your exploration could just begin with one plant that you have an affinity for. Anywhere that you find inspiration to create a ritual is great place to start.

What is important is that these rituals you create feel right for you in every aspect, even though they may be influenced by another culture; you feel able to create your own that honours your story and your heritage. Ultimately this can be more powerful, as you are bringing something uniquely yours to the ritual space, in turn this sows the seed for transformation and magic to happen.

Throughout the book I have included a few accounts from women who created their own rituals to help them integrate and honour their abortion. May these stories inspire you to delve into your own creativity, gather together the simple threads and begin to weave together a moment of honouring.

Aspects of ritual

1. Sacred space and time
   Creating the space and time for a ritual is the first powerful step on this journey. The space can be anywhere depending on the ritual; it is the commitment to dedicating your time to this act that makes the space potent. The transformation begins as soon as you commit to creating space for yourself, as you are stepping outside of your day-to-day world and entering into one where anything is possible.
2. Intention
   Having an intention is critical to any ritual, it is the intention that holds the power of transformation. When stating your intent, you are calling on the unseen realms to assist you in manifesting that intention. When deciding what you would like your intention to be, spend some time focusing on your heart and see what comes up. It may just be one word, or a whole stream of sentences. Try and keep the intent clear and concise, this will help in the resolution of the ritual.
3. Transformation
   Each ritual is a journey of transformation, regardless of what the ritual involves. During those minutes or hours that you are weaving the threads together, the shifts that can occur during a ritual may

happen on a multitude of levels, as you are entering a space where the old is falling away and the new is yet to be formed. This space of the in-between is potent, and not to be afraid of.

The transformation may not be tangible; it can manifest through a tiny, subtle shift in your energy, such as a new feeling of lightness around you, a deeper connection with your body or a sense of empowerment that you followed your intuition to create a meaningful ritual.

Each woman has her own unique timeline to healing from an abortion, so each transformation that takes place after a ritual will be different. An example of a transformation could be feeling a sense of peace when you place a small hand written note to the unborn child into the fire, its message to be delivered to the other side. Or it could happen several days after a ritual, when you realise that you are breathing deeply again for the first time.

These are examples of transformation taking place, each one as meaningful as the other. They are a sign that you are not quite the same person that you were at the beginning of this journey; a skin has been shed and you are moving towards a greater place of peace on this path of healing.

4. Gratitude

    Finally, gratitude. Gratitude is the essential fourth pillar of ritual. This way of giving thanks acknowledges all the parts that played a role in your ritual, both seen and unseen. In many of my rituals, I talk of giving thanks to any elements you have used from the earth. Whether it was soil, a stone, or some flowers, this all belongs to the earth and it is our responsibility to be grateful for that which we are given, therefore living in a circle of reciprocity. This may be a new concept for you. A stone cannot hear? Yet, the abundance of life surrounds us in all things! When we live with an intention to give back the blessings that we receive, we are immediately opening our hearts to receive immense love and healing.

An example of a simple ritual

An example of how we can elevate a mundane daily ritual to become a moment of peace and stillness is in the drinking of a cup of herbal tea. Instead of just drinking that cup of tea whilst doing a multitude of other activities, you could give yourself 15 minutes alone somewhere, to set the space. Your intention may be to get a good night's sleep, or to feel nourished by the herbs. The transformation is in the moment when you notice how the tea has influenced how you are feeling; are you feeling slightly calmer? Or more prepared for whatever the day brings?

Finally, offer gratitude for all that went into the making of your tea; for the water as the carrier for the herbs, for whoever gathered them from the earth that grew them and for all the elements that played their part in bringing you a delicious cup of tea. You may also wish to be grateful for choosing to stop your daily life and take this small window of time, just for yourself.

My own experience

My own experience of ritual stems from a desire to honour certain moments in my life that have felt very significant to me, despite the outside world not deeming them so—abortion is an example of such a moment. I felt an absence where my soul was yearning for an acknowledgement of what may have passed, so I created my own simple rituals, seeking to create sacred space where I could allow my feelings to surface and move through my body. With distant memories of lives lived where ritual was woven throughout the days and nights within communities and all of life was deemed sacred, I dug deep into my being to pull out these threads of memory, determined to see all parts of life's journey as worthy of a blessing.

Here is an account of how I created my own ritual to help me through the times of grief and loss.

> About a week after the abortion, I decided that I wanted to create a ritual to honour the loss and connect to the earth, so I went out and gathered some mud that I could mould into a little ball. I chose to select a few seeds to represent the cycle of earth returning again, I mixed these seeds and some dried rose petals into the ball of earth, carefully moulding it with my hands. Stepping out into the garden I asked where would be the most suitable place I can bury this little ball of life. I was guided towards a flower bed blooming with beautiful blue forget-me-nots. The name of the flower said it all. I sat at the edge of this flower bed and spoke to the flowers and the earth about why I had come, and may I bury this little bit of earth

that represents my loss, may the earth take care of it and may the new seeds sprout again in my life. I dug a small hole and placed the now dried mix of earth and seeds in it whilst whispering prayers of love and gratitude for the small being who rested in my body for such a small time. I felt held by the flowers, I felt that they were soothing both my spirit and the spirit of the foetus. Since that time whenever I see forget-me-nots I smile, and feel gladdened for this connection with these beautiful flowers and the little spirit baby that hovers nearby.

The rituals in this book

The rituals in this book are ones that have been created by myself and other women, through real experiences of what helped to acknowledge and heal from an abortion. If the concept of ritual is completely new to you, do not be afraid. You are fully capable of creating your own meaningful moment that will assist your healing in more ways than you can imagine. Ritual does not have to be "spiritual"; I have sought to include a whole variety of ways to honour an abortion. Some may seem so simple, yet the most important aspect is the *intention*, this transforms a regular action into a sacred one. As you look through them, your intuition will guide you to which ones, if any, you feel called to do. They are simply a framework for you to create your own rituals as you choose, equipping you with the tools that you need. My hope is that they are a resourceful platform to jump from, one that can inspire a desire to honour the loss and assist in your own journey through and after an abortion.

Before an abortion

Creating a simple ritual before an abortion can help prepare you for the inevitable loss. However, the challenging emotional states that you may be experiencing can make this a hard time to do a ritual. Any physical pregnancy symptoms too can make daily life feel like an uphill struggle. This is not a time to push yourself to do anything that you do not want to do, although I have included two possible rituals here, sometimes just making a delicious cup of tea is perfectly enough to imbue a sense of nourishment.

Writing a letter

This ritual came from a dear sister who created this with her partner. Although this can be a great way to involve your partner in the process, it will be equally transformative on your own.

Items needed:

- A piece of paper
- A quiet moment
- A safe place to burn paper, such as a fireplace, log burner, or a large metal saucepan

Ritual steps:

- On your piece of paper write a message to the one growing inside of you; how are you feeling? can you explain why you are going through with an abortion? if you could talk to it, what would you like to say? what are your fears or worries? Anything and everything can be written down, this is your chance to let go of what you may be holding back. If you are doing this with a partner, turn the piece of paper and hand it to him to repeat the exercise.
- Once you have both written the message, fold it up or put it in an envelope and place it into a fire, as the fire transforms your message think about your words reaching the baby. Fire embodies metamorphosis; opening a place of letting go of the old, as the piece of paper transforms into ash breathe out any fears and anxieties, the fire can help release all.
- Once you feel the ritual is complete, give thanks to the fire for the gift of the flame and all those who were present in helping you through this ritual.

The following account of a ritual demonstrates how with a few simple steps, a sacred moment can be created between two people who are choosing to honour the loss of a pregnancy.

> "My ritual with the burning of the note came from a friend. It was in the evening, I think between taking the first and second pill, I wrote a short message on a little piece of paper and my partner

wrote one on the back. Loving and kind, but also very brief and light. Then we burnt it over a candle together and let the message fly off into the universe."

—G.H.

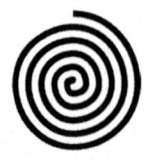

A bathing ritual

Taking a ritual bath is an act of profound self-care and healing for you, your body, and your spirit. A bath provides you with quiet space alone where you can connect with your womb and allow your mind to be still. I have already spoken about sacred bathing, so you can refer back to that in Chapter 2 for more information on the subject. Here I shall just give a brief outline of the actions to take to create this beautiful ceremony.

Items needed:

- A bath (if you don't have one, maybe a nearby friend could offer you theirs)
- A handful of dried flowers or/and suitable essential oils
- Candle(s)
- Incense if desired

Ritual steps:
Ensure that you have a window of time alone, this may be after the children have gone to bed, after dinner, it does not matter when. The most important thing is to communicate with those around you that you are taking a moment for yourself.

- Prepare the bathroom. A clean and clutter free space is important. Although clutter is subjective, as long as you can feel peaceful in your bathroom that is the most important consideration.

- Gather your materials.
- Start running the bath and light the candles, place them around the bath.
- Spending time away from artificial light is very beneficial for our nervous system, so once you have set up the candles, turn the lights off.
- Once the bath is run and the temperature right, place the dried or fresh flowers in the bath. Give thanks for the abundance of free flowing clean water that we have, and the gift of the flowers.
- Drop in your chosen essential oils and swirl the water around with your hands.
- *What is your intention?*
  Is it to nourish yourself? To calm your mind for 20 minutes? To mentally prepare for what is to come?
- Then step into the bath, and allow yourself to slowly give way to the water, surrendering to this moment that you have created.
- Soak for as long as you can/need to.
- Once you feel that you have finished bathing in the water, let the water out and imagine some of the difficult feelings that you may be going through going down the drain with the water. The water has washed you clear so you may step away feeling more peaceful and calm.
- Once out the bath, give thanks for giving yourself this gift of time and space.

You can repeat this ritual as often as you choose during the days and weeks, before and after.

After an abortion

I have separated the rituals into different sections depending on what the general theme is, helping you navigate your way to the ones that resonate most. The time frame when each woman chooses to honour her loss can vary hugely. For some they will feel ready days after an abortion, for others it may be many months before the time calls. These rituals are simply ideas for you to create your own rituals, in your own time.

A note on the full moon

The full moon is the peak moment of the month to release, let go and forgive all that you choose to. This window of lunar energy is extra-supportive of these actions, making it a perfect time to create ritual with some added lunar magic.

Herbal rituals

The following rituals involve the power of herbs to assist you in creating sacred space and holding a beautiful ritual of transformation.

Mugwort smoke bundle

The smoke of certain plants has been used as a healing and cleansing tool across the Earth for millennia. Mugwort is one such herb, its smoke is used to dispel negativity, increase awareness into other realms, and help to release trauma that is being held in the energy field around the body.

Mugwort is ruled by the planet Venus, a sign of its affinity with women. Mugwort's ability to increase dream time and help access parts of the unconscious also signifies a deep link with the Moon. As a plant ally, mugwort is there to assist you in healing your mind, body, and soul after an abortion.

When to do this ritual:
This ritual can be done at any moment after an abortion, whether that be days or decades. You can repeat it as often as you feel called to. Like any healing experience, there are many layers involved, so you may experience different sensations at different times.

Items needed:

- Dried mugwort (*Artemisia vulgaris*)
- Heatproof ceramic bowl

If you are one of the rare (and magical) women who always seem to have some dried mugwort stems hanging from your ceiling then you can skip this step. For everyone else, the first step is to go out and gather a couple of stems from a healthy living plant. If you are unsure of exactly what this plant looks like, take a good field guide, or a very knowledgeable friend with you before you head out on a mission to find this enchanting plant.

TIP: If you happen to see mugwort on a Full Moon night you may notice the silvery undersides to its leaves.

When you are certain you have come across a mugwort plant, ensure that there are several plants around so that you are not going to make an impact on a small wild population. Before you cut a few stems, introduce yourself to the plant and explain why you have come and what your intentions are. This builds a relationship of reciprocity with the plant, and acknowledges the unseen realms that we as well as the plants are immersed in.

Once you feel you are ready to gather a few stems, cut about 4 to 5 long stems. The length depends on how long you wish your bundle to be. No more than 30 cm will be needed. Before you leave, you may wish to make a small offering, thanking the plant for giving you some of her stems. This could be as simple as saying thank you to the plant, or even offering a pinch of dried lavender.

Next phase is to bunch the stems together and wrap some string around the bottom end. Find a place out of direct sunlight and well-aerated where you can hang the mugwort bundle. Leave to dry for several weeks.

NOTE—This ritual can be done alone, or you may wish to invite a plant loving friend to join you under the full moon as you go out gathering mugwort.

Intention:
To release and let go of any pain and sadness that surrounds my experience of abortion. I ask mugwort to bring healing to my womb, my body, and my spirit. Blessed be.

Ritual steps:

- Find a quiet peaceful space to be either alone or with a helper. Ensure there is a window that can be opened nearby to let the smoke out. Be wary of any smoke alarms that may go off. This can be done outside.
- Light a candle in front of you to focus on.
- State your intention aloud or silently.
- Either sitting or standing, light the mugwort bundle—you only want a small bit alight that you blow out immediately. There should be a

steady stream of smoke coming from the bundle. If it goes out, just relight it again to keep the smoke going.
- Once there is a steady stream of smoke, hold the bundle at arm's length away from your body and begin to move the smoke up and around you. Trust that the smoke travels to where it is most needed. You may find that you are focusing on a specific area, just allow the mugwort to direct you.
- The smoke can sometimes create a dreamy state, so sit down if you begin to feel wobbly.
- You may find yourself breathing deeply and letting go with your breath; the mugwort smoke will be working on many levels.
- Once you feel that it is complete. Place the mugwort bundle in the heatproof bowl, ensure that all the smoke stops burning, so that it is safe to put away later on.
- Spend a moment integrating how you are feeling. Finally give thanks to the mugwort.
- Drink some water to refresh yourself.
- Store the bundle somewhere safe, so that it is ready to be used again.

Planting new life

Items needed:

- A herb/plant/flower or even a tree that you love.
- A place in your garden or a pot.
- Some compost if planting in a pot.
- A sprinkle of water and some sunshine.

This simple but beautiful ritual connects you to the on-going spiral dance of life and death, within the natural world. There is an element of dedication to this ritual, you are dedicating your chosen plant to the life that was lost, therefore giving form to the invisible and creating new life to love.

Ritual steps:

- If the season is spring or summer, head out to a garden centre if possible and ask a member of staff to show which plants are perennial.

(this means although they will die back in winter, they will return to life come spring).
- Spend some time choosing the plant. It may be a small tree, a shrub, a herb, or simply a small flower. Try and choose one that you love, one that makes you feel joy when you look it at. If there are no flowers on the plant, then maybe find out if/when it flowers so you know what to look out for.

    NOTE—if it is winter, a solution would be to buy a house plant or hold the intention to go out and pick a plant when spring returns.
- Choose a suitable spot in your garden or on your patio/balcony for the plant.
- Give it a good water to help it adapt to its new home.
- Whether you are putting a plant in the earth or in your house, you are inviting this plant into your home. Maybe spend a few moments connecting with the plant, speaking about why you have bought this plant into your life and what it represents to you. Plants are as alive as we are, and they will listen to your story. Sometimes when we have feelings of grief, knowing that we have something to care for can bring a small but bright new purpose in our lives.
- Finally, give thanks for this plant in your life. May it fill your life with beauty.

Here is an account of a ritual, which was centred around a specific plant that offered connection to the loss of the abortion. This may inspire you to think about a plant or flower that feels connected to your loss. By cultivating a connection to this plant, you may nurture a lifelong and nourishing link to the loss of the pregnancy.

> "What came to mind was that at some point on Mother's Day violet called. It was African violet though. I had named the baby after my grandmother and she and I always cultivated these plants together. So I went, in deep grief, to the store around the corner and there was the most beautiful violet. She was the same colour as the baby's spirit. So she came home with me and it was something I could care for and put love into. Years later, also on Mother's Day, I went to gather violets in the forest and had a tremendous amount of grief surface. I made a tincture to work with which was immensely helpful."
> —H.S.

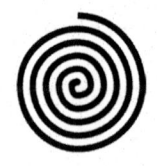

Vagina steam

Vagina steaming is an ancient way of using herbs to maintain a healthy female reproductive system. The moist heat of the steam softens the tissues of the vagina and acts as a potent carrier of the medicinal properties of the plants, which are absorbed into the tissues and directly enter the bloodstream.

It is a fantastic way to connect with your womb space, especially after going through something as traumatic as an abortion. Deciding to dedicate a window of time to yourself (and your womb) is a profound act of self-care, which opens the doors to healing any residual grief and trauma that may still be held within your body. This ritual is *only* to be done when you have stopped bleeding after the abortion.

Benefits of a vagina steam

- Increases circulation to the reproductive area.
- Offers a profound act of love towards your vagina and womb.
- Postpartum healing after an abortion or miscarriage, helping restore a connection with your womb.
- Increase in fertility.
- Emotional healing.

When not to have a vagina steam

- When menstruating or bleeding.
- If you have any wounds, sores, or blisters in the vagina area.
- If you have an infection.
- If you have a fever or are ill in any way.

Do NOT use essential oils, they are too strong to use for this purpose, stick to dried or fresh herbs.

How to have a vagina steam

Items needed:

- Either a slatted chair to let the steam pass through the chair or a *very* clean toilet (the latter is often easier and more readily available, and creates a private space). You can also now buy specifically created vagina steam chairs.
- Two large woollen blankets.
- A large heat proof glass bowl.
- Cup of dried or fresh herbs.

Ritual steps:

1. Make sure the toilet/chair and bathroom/space is clean. Maybe light a candle in there to create a warm inviting space.
2. Have a herbal tea or glass of water ready, maybe some calming music or a great book.
3. Simmer the herbs in a large saucepan filled with water for 5–10 minutes, then pour into the large heatproof bowl. Carry the bowl to the toilet where you then rest the bowl into the toilet.
4. Strip off your bottom half of clothes and underwear and sit down on the toilet, if the steam is too hot, allow it to cool slightly before you sit down. Only sit down when it feels comfortable for you. This is not meant to be painful, so really only sit when it feels like the right temperature.
5. Once sat, cover your entire lower half with one blanket, making a tent around the toilet to the ground, you want to trap the steam as much as possible.
6. Wrap the second blanket around your upper body, so that you stay warm.
7. Steam for 20–30 minutes.
8. Once complete, put on some warm clothes. Discard the herbal water, if possible outside, giving thanks to the Earth for the healing powers of the plants. If you can, either go to bed or lie down for an hour in warm clothes; resting is important to allow your body to complete the process.

Elemental rituals

The elements

In the following rituals we are working with one or more of the four elements: air, fire, water and earth. These pillars of our planet, balance and shape the world we live in, often reminding us of their unique power and strength. Each of the elements are represented as much in our own body as they are upon the earth, with each element corresponding to different parts of our body. Both of the oldest traditions of medicine; Traditional Chinese Medicine and Ayurvedic Medicine value the connection between good health and a balanced state of elements in the body.

Through learning a little more about how these four elements manifest on the earth and in our body, we can begin to see how interconnected we are with all of life. Our bodies are forever shifting and changing in relation to how these elemental forces are present in our surroundings. By working with the elements in ritual, we are inviting in the wisdom and strength of these elements to co-create a beautiful ritual of healing.

Air

Air is the element that exists all around us, yet is invisible to our eyes. We see how the air changes the shape of the clouds or moves through trees, and we feel its sensations upon our skin and moving in and out of our body.

The air is our breath, that which is essential for life and connects us to all the life around us. In the Ayurvedic tradition, air is called Vata (wind), and is primarily linked to the mind and the nervous system, which when out of balance is more susceptible to anxiety, stress and nervous conditions. When our own air element is balanced, we welcome in new ideas, new thoughts or beliefs into our lives. We breathe deeply, allowing life to move through us with each breath.

Fire

Fire provides the fuel for life to exist, it is the fire element that converts food to fuel, thus providing the energy for our bodies to function. The Sun represents the central focus of fire on this earth, yet the fire element is equally present in a small candle as it is an enormous forest fire. A central aspect to fire is transformation; this could be the food that is metabolised in our body to create energy, or the ability to transform creative sparks of inspiration into a tangible form.

When our fire element is imbalanced, we feel like our spark for life has gone, maybe we have a lacklustre appearance or more extreme we have lost the will to live. Our metabolism may be sluggish, and there is the need to withdraw from life. If there is an excess of fire, the skin may be very red, and we run our energy to the ground, lacking the balance to maintain a steady flow of life force.

When the fire element is balanced; our eyes are bright, we feel inspired by life and our body can easily digest food. We have a steady flow of energy, and are eager to fill our days with all that we love.

Water
The Water element includes all the natural forms of water including; lakes, rainstorms, snow and streams that flow across our planet. Within the body, water represents all that is fluid and flowing, from the blood to the tears. On a deeper level, the water element is our emotions.

An imbalanced water element manifests as fear, withholding of emotions, lack of feeling or love for self or others. From a physical perspective, a water imbalance may manifest as kidney problems or urinary tract infections.

When the water element is balanced within ourselves, we feel free to express ourselves fully, our heart is filled with compassion and empathy. We flow through life effortlessly, with the wisdom that water always finds a way around obstacles.

Earth
The Earth element is the solid ground we stand on, the layers of soil and rock that are the foundation for the rest of life to grow upon. Within our body, the earth element corresponds to our bones, our tissues, muscles, those solid forms for the oxygen(air) and the blood(water) to move through.

On an energetic level, the earth element represents how grounded we are, both in our body and on the earth. If it is unbalanced, we may feel stagnant or heavy in our body, unable to move through life freely. We feel stuck, as if it is always winter, with no desire to move forwards. Physically, this may manifest as constipation or digestion troubles, even problems with our bones or back, the structure of our body. If the earth element is balanced within us, we feel rooted, our body feels strong and solid, able to withstand the challenges of life with a calm and steady head.

Mixing your blood with the earth

Honouring the life that passed and seeding the new.

DISCLAIMER—This ritual is raw, earthy, and back to the elements.

Items needed:

- A few drops of your menstrual blood or a similar symbolic offering such as beetroot or cranberry juice.
- A small handful of earth.
- A place to bury this offering.
- A seed.

Ritual steps:

- This ritual is most suitable if you live in the countryside or wild place where you can peacefully be on your own and not be overlooked. One way to gather your own blood is to have your small handful of earth, or compost in your hands, head outside to a private place where you can squat down and hold the earth underneath (far enough away for there to be no chance of infection!) and allow the blood to fall onto the handful of earth.
- If you are doing this without real blood, then simply pour on some of the red liquid onto the earth handful. Once you feel there is sufficient blood, take the blood/earth into your hands and begin to mould into a ball, whisper your gratitude for your body, how she has the capacity to heal again, for the blood to return, for the foetus that left your body.
- Give thanks to the earth for holding you strong, for nourishing your body, and for giving life.
- Take the seed, it can be any seed, one from your kitchen or elsewhere. The act is only symbolic.
- Place the seed into this little ball in your hands, thanking the seed that represents *new life*, take a moment to consider what you would like to bring back to your life, maybe your monthly cycle, your freedom, or fertility.

- Hold this powerful symbol of old life mixed with new in your hands, and go find a place in nature where you can safely bury it into the ground.
- Finally give thanks for all the blessings you received in this ritual.

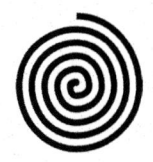

Giving to the waters

For this ritual you will need access to a coastal shore, or the banks of a flowing river. As women we have a special relationship with water; we are both the holders and creators of life on earth. Primarily yin in her essence, water teaches us how to flow with life, and move with grace past blocks and challenges on our path. Amongst some cultures, water is seen as the primordial Mother, making this element an ideal aspect of a ritual to honour a loss.

Even without doing a ritual, simply standing on the shore line in the presence of the waters can be immensely healing. Evidence suggests that the sound of the waves has been shown to increase the release of serotonin (the happy hormone) in the brain, and the salty sea air invigorates the energy around your body, leaving you feeling refreshed and revitalised.[35]

The essence of this ritual is to offer a token of your loss to the sea/the great oceans/rivers.

The waters are a place of regeneration; you may wish to see it as letting go of any pain connected to your experience and the loss of a little being. See the waters gather up this pain with gracious strength. Maybe you wish to ask that the waters keep the little soul safe until you feel the right moment for a baby. In your own time, find the words for your intention.

Below is an example of an intention that you may like to use. As ever, use the words that feel true to you and come from your heart.

Intention:
To release the feelings of [insert words] into these waters, so that they may be transformed and I may feel [insert words of how you would like to feel like]

Thank you sacred waters of this Earth.

Items needed:

- A stone: either one that you have collected from the beach or river side, or an old one you wish to use. Be sure to ask the river or the sea if you may take one of the stones, this does not need to be elaborate wording, and it may feel silly to ask an object that looks inanimate. However, this simple way of asking can be applied to anything that you may wish to gather from the earth. It is a way of honouring the fact that the elements of nature do not belong to us, but we have the power of speech to show our respect and love for all that the earth provides us.
- A quiet spot beside a body of water.

Ritual steps:

- Hold the stone in your hands and begin to think about everything you wish to let go of. When I say let go of, I am not expecting that any pain will suddenly disappear, it is more about letting go of the attachment to that pain. When this happens we can suddenly feel lighter as our burdens loosen their grip.
- As you hold that stone, send to it whatever you would like the water to take away; is it shame? fears of the future? anger?
- Imagine that this stone is filling up with all these feelings from your abortion that you no longer wish to feel. Choosing to acknowledge these feelings is a powerful step to letting them go.
- When you feel like you have said everything you wish to this stone, turn your attention to the water.
- State your intention, either aloud or in your head and throw the stone into the waters. This may be accompanied by sounds that you choose to make as you release these feelings to the water.
- Visualise the waters dissolving all that you put into your stone, taking them away and transforming them into light.

- Spend a few moments sitting quietly as you integrate this ritual. Do not underestimate these actions, this is big work.
- In whichever way feels comfortable for you, say thank you for this space by the water and for the transformations that occurred.
  Blessed be.

Writing rituals

Journaling

Journaling is a powerful practice that can help unlock and express emotions that you don't feel safe enough to express out loud but can allow to be written down. All you need is some paper and a pen. This is for your eyes only so just allow the words to come out. It could make no sense at all, it is a stream of consciousness on paper, giving an outlet to all kinds of thoughts/fears that you haven't been able to express in other forms.

Coloured pens and paint can also be helpful tools

A letter of forgiveness

Phase one

- Write a letter to the part of yourself that may be sad, angry, or hurt. Can you explain why you feel what you are feeling? Write as if you are writing to someone else, even though that other person is actually you. Imagine that you are sat opposite a friend who has gone through an abortion and is telling you how she is feeling. Yet you are that friend. Sometimes it is far easier to be kind and listen to others than it is to ourselves.
- Let the words flow on paper, until you feel that all you need to write in the moment has been written down. Thank yourself for the courage needed to express all that you did.
- The next step is to safely burn the letter, either in a fireplace or in a large metal container. The fire is an important part of this exercise; thanks to fire's capacity in transforming anger, sadness, or grief. As your letter burns focus on your words becoming ash. If you fancy, you could go and scatter the ash outside in gratitude for the elements.

Phase two
Next step is to write another letter to yourself, this time about all that you wish to attract into your life. Think of a barrel filled with muddy water, you have let that muddy water go into the earth, now you are filling it up with fresh clean water. This is what you are doing with the second letter, you are writing to yourself what you wish to fill yourself up with. It could be peace and acceptance about the experience. It could be forgiveness to yourself, or the foetus. It could be courage to step back into the world. There is a myriad of qualities that you may wish invite back into your life.

This letter is for you to keep somewhere safe, for you to re-read whenever you are struggling or feeling low. Use it as an anchor of strength for yourself.

Creative rituals

Something powerful happens when we put our heart and soul into a creative project, particularly one with intention. Here are a few ideas of creative rituals that may appeal to you. As always, see them as a frame for weaving in your own inspiration and ideas along the way.

A baking ritual

I owe a lot to cake. It has been a reliable source of income wherever I have lived, as I made my living baking all kinds of sweet goods and delivering them on the back of rickety bicycles. I often turn my hand to baking whenever I wish to feel soothed and nourished. There is such comfort to be found in going through the simple actions of combining a few ingredients, and then pulling something delicious out of the oven (hopefully).

This ritual is for all the cake lovers out there. If you are not a baker or have never baked a cake, why not invite a friend round to do some baking together and enjoy the deliciousness together.

Items needed:

- A recipe for the most indulgent delicious cake that you can imagine.
- Ingredients needed for said cake.
- Tunes to bake to.
- Fine company to help you eat the cake (or not).

The essence of this ritual is your *intention*.

Intention transforms this from just a regular baking of a cake, into a sacred few hours where you are creating something scrumptious to nourish you and your body.

Ritual steps:
As you begin to combine all the ingredients you need to make the cake, take a moment to think about your *intention*, how would you like to feel when eating this cake? nourished? You may choose to make it to say thanks to those that stood around you as you went through the abortion. The best time to speak your intent would be in the mixing and stirring of the batter, this in itself is an ancient way to imbue magic into something. As your stir with a spoon give thanks for all that has gone into make this cake, how would you like to feel when you eat this cake? how would you like others to feel? what are your thankful for? Finally, seal the stirring of the cake with the closing words of gratitude of your choosing. Put the cake in the oven for the time it needs. When ready, enjoy eating your delicious creation.

Making a womb bowl

This one is for those of you who love working with your hands, and find your stillest moments come when your hands are busy creating, allowing the rest of you to just be. The intention is to create a small bowl-shaped form that represents your womb. The form could be absolutely anything, any kind of shape; you may be surprised by what emerges from your hands. On a physiological level, our pelvis can be seen as a bowl, and our womb is held within that space. Once you have created a small womb bowl, it can serve as a way to communicate with your womb, you may wish to place small objects within it. Maybe a small crystal to represent the little being that your body held for a short time, or any other object to honour this space in your body.

This is a beautiful ritual to do together in a group of women, all making womb bowls together.

Items needed:

- Block of air dry clay (easily found online or in an art store).
- A clear and quiet space to sculpt.

Ritual steps:

- Firstly, choose how big you wish your bowl to be. Bear in mind that the smaller it is, the easier it will be to mould and the faster it dries.
- This technique is called "thumb bowls" or "pinch pots". Start by placing your thumb/finger into the middle of the ball of clay. Use this as the centre point and begin to press outwards, so that a loose shape of a bowl begins to form.
- The clay will help you decide the form, maybe it is a perfect circle, or more angular, or even wavy. Allow what comes, whilst holding the intention that this form represents your womb.
- If you choose, you can take a sharp object and carve into it with words or patterns.
- Once you feel it is complete, allow it to dry in accordance with the instructions for the clay you are using.
- Once dry, place somewhere special and enjoy your womb bowl.

This beautiful bathing ritual was kindly created by Lauren Rice who is a holistic skin therapist and the creator of Moonseed Rituals.

A ritual of release and self-love

What you will need:

– **Salts:** these can be any natural mineral salts such as Epsom, magnesium, Celtic or dead sea salts (not table salt).

Bathing in salt water has many wonderful benefits for the body, physically and spiritually. While salt water is healing and soothing on the skin, on an emotional and metaphysical level salts are often used for cleansing, detoxing negative energies, and purification. I like to use salts in many of my bath rituals that are focused on change and new beginnings.

– **Base oil:** it is important to distribute the essential oils in a protective base oil so they don't irritate the skin, this can be as simple as virgin olive oil or a nourishing plant oil like borage or grapeseed oil.

– **Essential oils:** the key element to this bath are the essential oils chosen for the blend and the effect they have on the body and mind. The most important thing is to choose oils which you are personally attracted to and enjoy the scent, but for this recipe I have listed several oils because of their heart healing benefits.

- **Sweet orange:** uplifting, mood stimulant.
- **Geranium:** balances hormones, antidepressant, mood stimulant.
- **Jasmine:** a valuable oil for all areas of reproductive health. Antidepressant and anti-anxiolytic effects, emotionally warming.
- **Rose:** considered to be governed by Venus, rose oil has been used in all matters of female reproduction, physically and emotionally. Supports those in grief and aids heart healing.
- **Chamomile:** calming and soothing effects on the emotions, an antidepressant.
- **Herbs:** I have chosen two herbs for their connection with women and the heart.
- **Rose petals:** the ultimate heart healing herb, rose has been used alongside woman's healing remedies for centuries. On an energetic level, rose is known to connect the heart to the womb, concentrating love in an area that often holds trauma and shame.
- **Motherwort:** the name motherwort indicated this plant's useful quality for many women's conditions and is often considered the "wise woman" of herbs. She is known to build courage and to heal a wounded heart.
- **Crystal** (optional): rose quartz has a direct link with heart energy and encourages unconditional self-love.
- **Tools:** mixing bowl, candles, music.

Bathing ritual

Begin this ritual by blending up your bath potion. This should consist of salt, a base oil, essential oils and herbs. First fill a bowl with your chosen salt and in a separate bowl mix together two teaspoons of your base oil along with 6 drops of essential oil. Give everything a good mix so the oil is distributed well with the salt and then begin to add your desired amount of herbs. It really is your choice as to how much herbal mixture you would like to bathe in. Once the mixture is prepared, I like to pour it into a decorative bowl and place it by the bath next to the candles and crystals while the tub fills.

While you run the bath, place a few candles around the room and play some beautiful, relaxing music. Once the bath is ready, pour a generous amount of the mixture into the bath water and submerge your body. You can either place the rose quartz directly in the bath or keep it on the side. During this time, you are to just switch off and relax, allow the salt, herbs, oils, and crystal to do their work. Deep inhalations of the diffused essential oils will bring about a relaxation response and the most important thing is that you allow some time for your mind to quieten down and for your body to release tension.

If any emotions come up during this time, allow them to flow out of you and imagine them soaking into the water where, when you finally step out and drain away the bath water they will flow away down the drain, leaving only peace and pure love behind.

If you don't have a bath, this ritual can still be done in the shower or as a foot bath. For the shower you can still use the candles and music and you will need to add the ritual blend into a cotton bag or muslin cloth that you can tie around the shower head to the water can run through it and allow the salts, oils and herbs to be released with the water and steam. If you prefer to have a foot bath, the mixture can be poured into a large bowl or basin of warm water and allow your feet to soak for at least 15 minutes.

After a bath ritual, gather up the herbs before they go down the drain, place them back in the bowl and when you get the chance, return them back to the earth and give thanks for their healing and comfort.

CHAPTER 6

Nutrition

How we nourish our bodies affects not only our physical health but our mental and emotional wellbeing too. When our body is fit, vital, and radiant in health there is a far greater capacity to heal from any illnesses, traumatic events, or stress that we may experience. When we eat delicious healthy food we are sending a sign to our bodies that we love and care for them and they will respond by giving us energy and strength to live well.

I am writing a small amount on this topic of nutrition for the following reasons:

- What we eat has a direct impact on our health. Food is medicine.
- Cooking delicious meals is an empowering act in healing your body.
- The after effects of an abortion may lessen when we increase the consumption of certain foods—e.g. iron rich foods help maintain energy levels during the loss of blood.
- Chocolate (cacao) can be instrumental to healing after an abortion.

Essential vitamins and minerals we need as women

Whilst functionally men and women may have many similarities, our hormonal and physiological differences require particular nutritional needs. A significant aspect of this difference is that a woman's' body (in most cases) has a menstrual cycle, during which they lose up to 80 ml of blood each month, resulting in a monthly loss of essential minerals. By ensuring that we have a healthy diet rich in certain foods, our body is able to maintain a balanced level of health and energy throughout the month.

Below I list a couple of the most important minerals that we need; however, this is by no means a comprehensive list. If you are curious to further your interest in nutrition for women's health, I include a couple of sources at the back of the book for you to peruse.

Iron

Iron is essential for the production of haemoglobin, which is the substance that allows our red blood cells to carry oxygen. When a body is low in iron, there is insufficient haemoglobin to transport oxygen to all the organs, muscles, and tissues, which can result in fatigue amongst other symptoms. Women need far more iron than men to maintain a healthy body, due to menstruation and pregnancy.[36]

Natural sources of iron include:

– Red meat
– Leafy greens such as spinach, kale, spring greens
– Blackstrap molasses
– Beetroot
– Dried figs
– Pulses and beans such as red lentils, chickpeas, kidney beans.

NB: It is possible to maintain high iron levels without eating meat.

Why is it important to have enough iron in your diet post-abortion?

During menstruation the body is losing several tablespoons of blood, depending on how heavy or light the flow is. However, after an abortion, especially if it is The Pill Method, the body will be releasing more blood and tissue than normal, therefore affecting the iron levels more than a normal period. After a surgical abortion there could be less bleeding as the foetus has been removed during surgery; however, each body and womb reacts differently to the procedure, there is no normal. Symptoms of iron deficiency can vary; common ones are fatigue, pale skin, and heart palpitations.[37] If you are still bleeding several weeks after then it is extra important to nourish yourself with some of these iron rich foods; this will speed up your healing process and help you to regain your strength again.

A note on supplements

When we eat a healthy and balanced diet, our body is constantly extracting all the minerals and nutrients that it needs from the foods. Supplements can be useful if we discover that the body has particularly low levels of a certain mineral or vitamin. However, despite having a high content of a particular nutrient, supplements are by no means a substitute for eating delicious healthy seasonal food. When we eat spinach or kale, for example, not only are we absorbing a high amount of iron, but also an array of other minerals, such as vitamins C and K, therefore nourishing the body in a multitude of ways. However, due to the intensive farming practice in today's world, the soil is severely depleted in nutrients, which has subsequently resulted in foods that are less rich in nutritional value. This can be a good reason to include certain well-sourced supplements in your diet. It is always worth doing some research before you enter into the vast world of supplements.

Nettle miso broth

Here is an iron rich recipe perfect for spring when the nettles are abundant across the land. If you are not able to access nettles, feel free to substitute them for other leafy greens such as kale or chard.

Nettles are packed full of nutrients and minerals, including iron, magnesium, and vitamin C, amongst many others. When we eat wild foods in tune with the seasons we are nourishing our body on multiple levels, helping align our bodies with the earth's cycles.

In spring you are likely to see an abundance of nettles and dandelions on any green patch of land. It is no coincidence that these plants that aid the body in detoxifying and cleansing arrive just when we need them. Spring is the time when our livers are active, working to cleanse our systems from the excess of winter, and we can help our bodies in doing their work by incorporating some of these healing wild foods into our diet.

*Foraging note—If you are able to harvest nettles, collect only the top part of the plant, gather where there has been no chemical spraying or car pollution, and be sure to gather sustainably; take only what you need and leave the rest for other foragers and wildlife.

Miso is made from fermented soybeans. It is rich in iron, potassium, and calcium, making this delicious Japanese import a great addition to your meals.

Ingredients

- A large handful of fresh nettle tops (be sure to give them a shake once harvested so any little creatures fall off)
- Olive or coconut
- Garlic
- 1 onion
- Optional extras—broccoli, kale, spring greens, spinach.

Method

Heat the oil in a saucepan. When hot, add a chopped onion and a crushed garlic clove, allow to gently soften for 5 minutes stirring all the time. Once soft, add the handful of nettles and any greens that you fancy. Stir so that they are mixed in with the onions and garlic. Add some stock, if its just for one, pour enough so that is a good inch or two over the nettles and onions. Bring to the boil, then simmer for 15 minutes. Once the nettles have broken down and reduced in size and any veg you added is soft, stir in a good tablespoon of miso, a pinch of salt and pepper, and a squeeze of lemon. Pour into a bowl and enjoy.

Magnesium

One of the roles of magnesium in the body is to retain normal nerve and muscle function. Women who have lower levels of magnesium in their bodies can be prone to menstrual cramps and headaches during the pre-menstrual phase of their cycle. This essential nutrient also assists in rebuilding tissues in the body, which is why magnesium plays such a critical role in pregnancy. During those months the body is rapidly growing a foetus, putting much of its energy into this process. Despite no longer being pregnant, magnesium can assist the uterus in rebuilding the endometrial lining again in preparation for the return of your menstrual cycle.

Magnesium rich foods:

- Bananas
- Cacao
- Sesame seeds
- Pumpkin seeds
- Chard/spinach

Cacao

Chocolate is a lifelong love affair for many women, and there is actual scientific proof that validates our need for chocolate! This is due to the high levels of magnesium in cacao (the raw product of cocoa beans), which does mean that the higher percentage of chocolate the more magnesium goodness you will receive.

Cacao is the raw form of chocolate; this is different to cocoa which is the processed form of cacao beans. In short, a milky Dairy Milk does not have much cacao compared to a Green and Blacks 80% bar.

Benefits of high percentage chocolate/raw cacao powder:

- Mood enhancing by increasing serotonin (the happy hormone)
- Enhances energy
- Increase of love for self and others, thanks to cacao's affinity with the heart chakra.

Divine hot chocolate

You will need:

- Any milk of your choice.
- Raw/normal cacao powder

- Spice options: cinnamon, turmeric, cardamom, saffron, ashwagandha, cayenne.
- For extra chocolate—several squares of dark chocolate.

Fill the cup that you are drinking your hot choc in with milk, and pour this into a pan. Gently turn the heat up. NB: depending on how creamy you want your hot choc, you can either use just milk or half it with some water to make it slightly less rich. Add in 1–2 large teaspoons of cocoa powder and a pinch of spices, if using. **Caution:** you only need the tiniest sprinkle of cayenne. Drop a few squares of your favourite dark chocolate and start stirring with a whisk to help the chocolate melt and the spices to infuse. Don't let the milk boil, instead just heat gently until it reaches a perfect temperature for you. Pour into a mug and enjoy.

Beetroot and chocolate cake

(Inspired by green kitchen stories)

This cake has the double whammy of magnesium filled cocoa powder and mineral rich beetroot. I have renamed this cake—The Period Cake—due to the countless times I have baked it on the first day I bleed.

The beetroot makes the cake rich and earthy along with a fantastic purple colour.

Ingredients

- 110 g oil (olive or coconut)
- 125 ml of maple syrup/agave/runny honey
- 60 g dark chocolate for melting
- 50 g dark chocolate for breaking into chunks.
- A couple of medium sized beetroots, around 225 g grated.
- 3 eggs
- 200 g plain or spelt flour
- 2 tsp baking powder
- 35 g cocoa powder (raw if possible)
- A pinch of sea salt
- A small teaspoon of ground cardamom
- A tablespoon of sesame seeds.

Method

Pre-heat the oven to 180°C/160°C (fan). Start by combining the oil, 60 g chocolate and maple syrup in a pan and very gently heating until just melted. Grate the beetroot and combine to the chocolate/oil mix. Whisk the eggs in a separate bowl, then add to the beetroot mix. In a separate bowl, mix all the dry ingredients together with a whisk or fork to dissolve any baking powder lumps. Finally combine the wet and dry ingredients together and add in the 50 g of broken up bits of chocolate. Stir everything until combined into a delicious looking red chocolate mix. Line a loaf tin with baking parchment and pour the mix into the tin, sprinkle with a few sesame seeds. Pop into the oven and bake for around 40 minutes. You will know that it is ready when the cake has risen, the top has slightly cracked, and when you stick a knife in it comes out mostly clean. As the cake is quite moist, do not be concerned if there is some mixture that sticks to the knife. Leave to cool for as long as you can. Enjoy.

Hormones and seeds

Another way to help re-establish balance in your body and hormones after an abortion is to include a daily dose of certain seeds. After an abortion, the hormones are in a state of shock as our body has shifted from a pregnant state to a not pregnant state, often in a matter of hours. This sudden drop in hormones can have a dramatic impact on the emotions in the days and weeks after.

Including these seeds into your diet is an easy way to help normalise your hormones, assist the menstrual cycle, and nourish your health. In recent years there has been talk of "seed cycling"; this involves eating different seeds at different times of your menstrual cycle. Whilst this may also be effective, it can prove to be too much of a hassle for some women, and by simply just including a daily dose of seeds is enough to receive many of their healing benefits.

One of the benefits of including seeds into your daily diet is to stabilise levels of oestrogen and progesterone, the key hormones of the menstrual cycle. By maintaining optimal hormonal levels, the common symptoms of migraines, breast tenderness, and mood swings can be avoided. Often when there are symptoms of hormonal imbalance in the body this is due to excess oestrogen and one of the main actions of these seeds is to help the body metabolise the oestrogen, therefore creating a more balanced hormonal state.

Which seeds?

Flax seeds (Linseeds)

These humble brown seeds from the ancient flax plant contain a multitude of essential vitamins and nutrients. Primarily lignans, which contain antioxidant compounds and phyto-oestrogens that assist in balancing the hormones.[38] Flax seeds also contain a high amount of fibre, which aids regular bowel movement, allowing the body to metabolise excess oestrogen to maintain a balanced hormonal state.

They are best consumed in their ground form; you can either buy ready-ground or just grind a few spoons in a coffee or spice grinder.

Pumpkin seeds

Pumpkin seeds are packed full of zinc and magnesium. They are also rich in omega 3s, which help the blood flow to the uterus, increase progesterone secretion, and rebuild cell membranes.[39]

Sunflower seeds

High in the trace mineral selenium, which research suggests supports oestrogen detoxification in the liver therefore reducing excess oestrogen in the body. Signs of high levels of oestrogen include breast tenderness before menstruation, fibroids, and intense irritability during the premenstrual phase.[40]

Sesame seeds

These seeds are rich in magnesium, copper, and zinc, all contributing to the health of the bones, skin, and respiratory system. They are also a great source of fibre in the diet.[41]

How many seeds to take?

Generally, a 1–2 tablespoon size of any of the seeds above is a great way to include them in your daily diet. Ways to include them could be adding them to your breakfast porridge, sprinkle them on salads, or just toast them and snack on them throughout the day.

CHAPTER 7

Body, movement and voice practices

Creating space in your life for an embodied practice can play a key role in healing from an abortion. The experience of pregnancy is physical; it is rooted in our wombs and our bodies. When we halt that natural process, it is our wombs that feel the loss and hold the trauma of the experience. By engaging in physical movement, we are opening up a space for those memories within the womb to move through our bodies and be released. These practices help to get us out of our minds, therefore tuning into the wisdom of our bodies and encouraging the healing energy to flow.

Over the next few pages I describe a few of these practices; you could view them as tools to use in the months or years after an abortion for moments for when you feel stuck in certain emotional states and are seeking a way to move through difficult times. The more tools that we have to help us ground, release, and move, the easier it is to build up our strength and feel ready to face all that we need to.

Yoga

Yoga is an ancient form of meditative movement practice originating in India. Within the movements there is a strong focus on the breath, this helps to reduce mental chatter and brings you back into the present moment with your body.

These poses are especially helpful for women after an abortion when it is best to avoid intense exercise and movement. They encourage us to return to our breath with a focus on grounding back in the body and rebalancing the nervous system. They can be done in a sequence or simply on their own, as and when you have a spare moment to be still.

Items needed: you will either need a block or bolster or several cushions and folded blankets. It will be worth taking the time for the preparation, for the deep rest that comes from these poses.

My gratitude for these yoga poses goes to qualified Restorative Yoga Teacher Heather Sanderson.

1. Legs up the wall—this will help to ground and allow energy to return to your body, if needed.

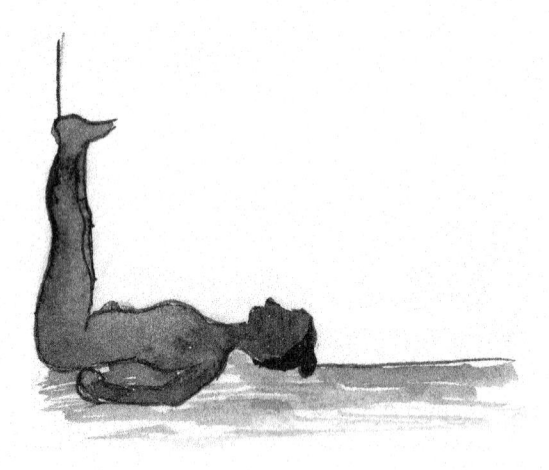

2. Supported wheel (with a pillow or two or a bolster under the knees, feet touching the ground or on blocks, and a rolled firm blanket under the bottom of the shoulder blade of any comfortable height). A gentle opening of the heart and overall support of the nervous system.

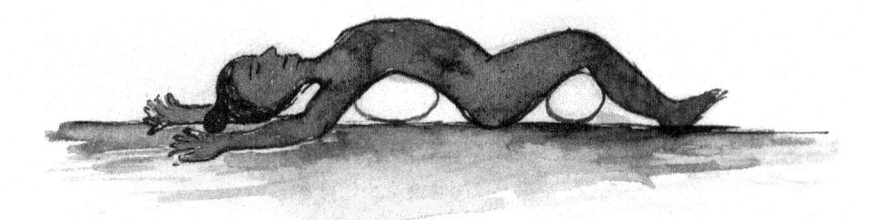

3. Supported goddess pose (with a cushion or a bolster on an angle supported by blocks. You rest back with your palms open and facing up, legs in a diamond with a blanket roll or blocks supported the knees). A gentle opening of the pelvic bowl and hips, supported heart.

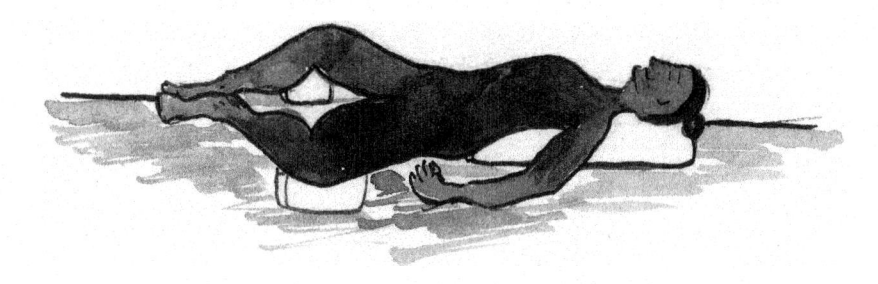

4. Supported bridge (with a block at the sacrum) A supported way to bring energy to the womb while opening the heart and circulating energy into the ground.

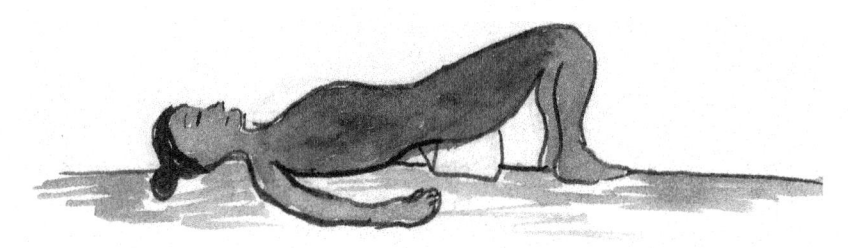

5. Side shavasana (resting on the right side holding a pillow or bolster at your heart, resting your head on it, with another between the knees). A way to rest and integrate energy. Holding onto a pillow or bolster also allows for any grief to flow, if needed.

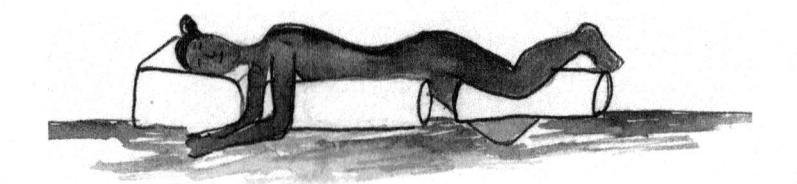

Dance

Our bodies hold the memory of everything that has ever happened to them within their cells. This means that traumatic memories can be stuck within our body for many years until we seek healing or engage in practices to help release them. Dance is one such practice that is a fantastic and liberating way to let go, shake off, and move through challenging times in our lives. Dancing in any form is great; from going wild in your room to music, going to an organised dance class, or trying out a form of free movement, such as 5-Rhythm class (more information in the Resources at the back of the book.)

Grounding to the earth

For this exercise you will need a garden or a calm spot in the local park. Simply lie on the earth, either face up or face down and with a deep breath imagine letting go of all the tension in your body. Spend some minutes feeling the support of the soil beneath you, imagine that the earth is taking away all of your worries and sadness.

In recent years the act of "grounding" has been proven to dramatically reduce nervous tension and stress in the body.[42] If you would rather not lie on the earth, then simply take off your shoes and socks and spend a few minutes grounding in this way with your bare feet on the soil. Our feet act as the receptors to the energy of the earth and instantly bring a sense of calm to the body and nervous system.

This grounding practice is useful to do whenever life gets too much. The restorative power of nature can never be underestimated, it is a space that we all have access to and can be immensely helpful in coping with the demands of modern day life.

The earth has the capacity to transmute what we want to let go of, she is there to hold you and take in the pain you are feeling. If you feel alone after an abortion, why not take a walk and find a tree that calls to you. Try sitting with this tree for some time, maybe even starting a conversation, explaining why you are seeking support. Observe how you feel as your back rests against the trunk, as you breath in the air around you. When you choose to leave, observe again if you feel differently and give thanks to the tree.

Voice

Women have used song to mark and honour moments of change, trauma, and transition since the beginning of time. Our voice represents how we express ourselves in the world; we are creating through our voice. When we have experienced challenging moments of shame, trauma or grief, we can develop a block in our voices; this is particularly relevant to the taboo of abortion where very little is spoken openly about the experience. There is a history of women's voices being repressed throughout time, although our voices are beginning to be honoured and heard in many more ways, we still have a long path ahead of us.

The first step to healing is through our own relationship with our voice. What wants to be released through our voice? (without it being directed at someone).

If after an abortion you begin to notice feelings of anger that were not expressed or other feelings that you would like to express, then here are few options you may choose to take. Be gentle with yourself especially if you are only in the recent aftermath of an abortion.

- Put on your headphones and sing loudly to your favourite music.
- If you live near the sea, head down there on a stormy day and allow the waves and wind to carry your voice away.
- Find a friend who is open to sharing this voice releasing experience with you, and can also support you if needs be. Choose as remote a location as possible, with few people around (I first did this in a large park in the city on a windy day).

  Stand back to back with your friend, feel the support of each other and begin to allow your voice to emerge, maybe you scream or hum or shout. It doesn't matter, your voice will take over and just allow those sounds to come out. Hold the intention to let go of anything that may be blocking you from being your best self. Allow the process to continue until you feel the natural moment to return to silence. If this exercise has released any emotions, take the time to be present with how you are feeling and connect to the support of your friends back behind you. It is important to take a few deep breaths here and feel the support of the earth under your feet as you integrate any changes that you may feel. This exercise can release some significant emotions. Once you feel complete, you can each turn around and give each other a hug to close this moment you shared.

CHAPTER 8

Boyfriends, partners, husbands

To all the men out there who stand next to their girlfriends, partners, wives, and friends whilst they go through an abortion, I am writing this for you. You will never go through an abortion and you have no idea what it feels like, but there are ways that you can support, love, and hold a woman who is or has gone through one. If you are the father of the foetus that is going to be leaving your partner's body, then an abortion can be deeply moving and sad for you as well as the woman. You are one half of this little being, a co-creation between you and your partner, and maybe you are distressed by their decision to have an abortion. Even though you are not the one who is pregnant, you have every right to feel sadness in this decision.

There may be certain men who are against their partner having an abortion, this is a challenging dynamic for both the man and the woman to be in, as it is the woman's body and is ultimately her choice at the end of the day. However, if you do feel strongly against your partner ending the pregnancy, then I encourage you to sit down and communicate how you feel, your thoughts about the decision are also valid. This will help resolve any feelings of powerlessness that may be arising, and could open up a space for you to hear how she is truly feeling, and why she feels that this is the best decision.

An important factor in journeying through this time together is to understand why there is a desire for an abortion; it may be in the best interests of your relationship and/or family, the timing may be wrong, she may be afraid, amongst countless other reasons. By truly coming to accept and respect her choice, you open up a safe space for her emotions to flow, encouraging her feelings to evolve, and ultimately promote honest communication.

Support for men

The impact that an abortion can have on men is rarely acknowledged within both relationships and society. This is for the obvious reason that it is the woman who is going through the ordeal, and men may be on the receiving end of anger and blame. There are numerous reasons and ways that women go through abortions, and some men are part of their journey, however many are not. I am choosing to offer support for the men who felt a deep sense of loss after the experience, even if they were not present.

Men's emotions are rarely given the space that they deserve within the patriarchal model of today's society, this has resulted in a deep imprint upon men's psyche's that it is weak or soft to show how they are feeling. Although this is subtly shifting for some, with the increase of men's groups, both men and women have a long way to come before we can give space to all that wants to be heard from the masculine perspective.

What can men do to support themselves?

- **Sit with how you are feeling.** This may sound too simple, but for some men it may be a challenging or new task, as difficult to face emotions may normally be swept underneath the carpet. Sitting with how you are feeling could take many forms; it may be spending some time alone in the garden, or going for a walk alone, or even talking to a close trusted male friend about your feelings. The crucial element is that you are giving space for anything that you may have felt following a close experience with an abortion to emerge. This is brave work, if at any point this becomes an overwhelming task, then seek professional counselling from someone who you can trust.

- **Take time out for yourself.** If you are in a partnership with a woman who recently went through an abortion, the weeks following may be fraught as her hormones begin to rebalance and she adjusts to the loss of what just happened. As present as you may be for her, it is equally important for you to support yourself during this time, especially if you are feeling any grief or sadness. If you are in a partnership with someone, it is important to communicate that you need some time for yourself, gently explain why this is so that she does not feel rejected or lost without you. You may find that when you take time out for yourself, you are also allowing yourself to feel how the abortion has impacted you for the first time. By facing these emotions head on, you are beginning to take responsibility for how you are feeling. This allows for a deeper integration of the experience, and as these emotions move through you, you may notice a feeling of spaciousness or peace begin to emerge. This is a sign that you are on the path of authentically healing from the experience, and becoming more attune to your inner self.

- **Honest communication.** This is both with yourself and your partner. If you really wanted this baby, however your partner chose otherwise, then it is important that you honour your feelings about her decision. Maybe you are feeling resentment or anger or grief towards her. This is all okay. Even by realising that you feel angry is an enormous step in the direction of healing from this pain. What is important, is that you have ways or your find ways to move through the tender state that you are in. Do not take it out on her, she is on her own journey of recovery. However, you may feel that you are in a strong enough partnership to travel this path of healing from an abortion together, in which case, remain mindful of how much support she can give.

- **Honour the grief.** Grief can creep up on you in mysterious ways and in the strangest of places. For some, the grief may not be immediate, but could manifest as a prolonged depressed state, or for others it may be confused with rage or blame for oneself. The process of healing from this experience takes time, and each man will move through this journey on his own unique timeline. Bear in mind, that when grief is felt, you may be tapping into the deep wells of unexpressed grief across generations of men who felt that they were not able to express their emotions. From this perspective, we can appreciate how courageous it is when men give themselves permission to cry and grieve for all their losses. May us women, support you in this work.

- **Create a simple ritual.** Creating a ritual can be the simplest of acts, and a powerful way to honour the loss. A ritual could be planting a tree, or writing a poem, or simply finding a special piece of wood or stone that you feel could represent the loss you feel. There are no rules, only for you to follow a calling to mark the experience in a symbolic way. If you have never created a ritual before then I suggest you read the chapter on rituals to give you some ideas.

- **Seek help from a professional counsellor.** If you are in a partnership with a woman who has gone through an abortion, she may not be in a good space to be able to support you as you process your own emotions. By seeking external support, this can take pressure off the relationship, and give you the chance to feel heard and seen for all that you are going through.

In time, you will be able to reflect upon this experience, and see where your life has evolved as a result of this journey that you made alone, or with someone. Maybe, going through this journey with a loved one has made you realise how much you would like to be a father one day. Or, this experience could have highlighted an area of your relationship that needs some care and attention. Regardless of your reflections, I hope that you are able to honour your own loss of the little being in the time and space that feels right for you, with all the support you need.

Herbs to support men

During the days or weeks that surround an abortion, it can make a real difference if you have as many tools to support yourself as you can. The inclusion of herbal medicine in this time can have a positive impact on how you feel both physically and emotionally. Not only will the herbs nourish you, but if you are the partner of a woman who has recently ended a pregnancy, having a very basic knowledge of herbal teas that you could make for her is a lovely way to be able to offer support.

As you read through the list of herbs, see if there are one or two that jump out at you. If this happens, this means that your body felt a resonance with that herb and it is likely to be one that can support you. If you feel indifferent to the herbs, then there are a number of factors that can help you choose one or two:

- Are any of them growing in your garden?
- Have you tried one of them before and really like the taste?
- Does the description of the herb feel aligned to how you are feeling?

Why take herbal medicine?

Through consciously choosing to drink a cup of herbal tea each day, you are giving yourself a small precious moment of time to care for how you are feeling. Even if you only have 10 minutes spare, or you have the space to fill a flask with a herbal brew and take a walk, the time is irrelevant, as it is the intention to tend to yourself that counts. If you are completely new to the realm of herbal medicine, try approaching it with a beginner's mind, filled with curiosity. Each herb tastes completely different to the next and offers many healing properties. If you are lucky enough to live near wild corners where plants grow freely, I encourage you to explore with a good field guide—to see if any of these plants are medicinal and whether their properties are supportive for how you are feeling.

How to take the herbs?

The simplest way to take the following herbs is to make a herbal tea. You can either take them on their own, or mix a couple together—you cannot go wrong. The worst that will happen is you make a herbal tea that is too strong and you can't drink it. Experiment with different herbs to find which ones you like, and feel how they affect your body and mind. To find out more about how to make a herbal tea, please head to the chapter on Herbal Medicine for details on the method and dosage.

This is only a small selection from many herbs that could be of support to you during this time. I have sought to include ones that I have found to be strengthening and soothing to the body during challenging times in life.

Hawthorn

Crataegus monogyna

Hawthorn is often used as a medicine for the heart, both physically and emotionally. The leaves, flowers, and berries are safe and effective to take for any kinds of grief or trauma that you have experienced. If it is the season, you can go out and gather some hawthorn flowers or berries to make a herbal tea with, even the simple act of foraging these beautiful flowers can lighten the spirits.

Sage

Salvia officinalis

Sage is a wonderful herb to take when you feel depleted of energy, this may be the result of emotional strain or physical illness. The origin of its Latin name *'Salvia'* means 'to save', showing how valued it was as a herb to heal people's ills. If you are struggling for energy and wonder where your strength to face challenging situations have gone, then try drinking one or several cups of sage tea for a few days until you feel restored.

Rosemary

Rosmarinus officinalis

Rosemary is a highly aromatic herb that can stimulate the mind and ease lethargy. With a strong connection to the sun, and the element of fire, rosemary is best taken when you are lacking in energy or internal fire. When life feels grey and you need a boost of fire back into your life, make a rosemary tea; Or, if you have some, place a few drops of rosemary essential oil on a tissue and inhale deeply through your nose.

Nettle

Urtica dioica

Nettle is an all-round tonic, that strengthens and supports the body. Nettle could be useful to take if you find yourself run down both emotionally and physically after supporting someone through an abortion. Nettle will work to bring back vitality to your body, and ensure that you have all the strength you need to navigate the following weeks or months. If it is spring, and you know a good and clean source of nettles, you may wish to experiment with cooking or steaming them, which is another great way to include them in your diet.

Oat straw

Avena sativa

Oat straw is a restorative herb that rebalances the adrenal glands after times of stress and anxiety. A nourishing and mineral rich herb, it can be liberally drunk as a herbal tea during tense and fraught times. To make a really soothing herbal tea, you could combine it with chamomile and skullcap.

Skullcap

Scutellaria lateriflora

Skullcap is a nourishing nervine, which means it reduces the impact of stress on the body and calms the mind. If you find your mind to be overactive and filled with anxiety about the abortion, this herb would make an excellent tea to take before bed, encouraging sleep to come more easily. Equally, if you are supporting a woman through an abortion, you could make a big flask of this tea to take with you to the clinic, which you could both drink before and after, to gently encourage a state of calm during this tense time.

Ways to support a woman going through an abortion

Any support that you can give your partner before, during and after an abortion will be valued. However, it is important to be conscious of your own capacity to give at this time, in terms of energy and emotional support. How can you ensure that you are looking after yourself too?

By checking in with how you are feeling, and taking care of your own needs as well has hers, you will find your capacity to offer support is far greater as a result. This is a tough time for both of you, but, by honouring what is coming up for you and releasing any pressure to be the perfect partner, then you are in the best position to help guide your partner through this journey.

I have given a few tips to how you may support her. I hope you find this a short helpful guide to supporting her through this journey with all your love and compassion.

Before the abortion—This is a tense and fraught time. She will need support, reassurance, and hugs from you. Her hormones and consequently her emotions will be like a pendulum, try not to take anything personally. This all will pass.

After the abortion—Be the tea-maker, hot water bottle filler and all-round giver of love. This is the time to listen; to her words, her body language—is it saying she wants sex or not. Maybe all she needs is gentle intimate time together. Penetrative sex is not a good idea whilst her body is bleeding, allow her body time to rebalance and heal. She may simply want to be held, this is enough.

One more thing, it is extremely easy for a woman to get pregnant straight after an abortion as her body naturally wants to replace what was lost. If as a couple you have decided that you would not like to get pregnant in the following months, then it is up to you to be responsible for this as much as her. Against all my rationality, there was a part of me that wanted to get pregnant straight away, when really I did not at all. I spoke to my partner about this and asked him to gently remind me of this from time to time when in the heat of the moment.

As the weeks and months pass, time begins to heal an abortion, however, this is not to say that it must never be spoken about. This also applies to friends and female partners of a woman who has gone through one. After the initial period of time, abortions are often rarely spoken about, even amongst the closest of girlfriends! If you are in a relationship and went through one together then I invite you once in a while to ask her: How she is feeling? Does she want to talk about it? Does she feel the presence of the little being that left her body? This recognition of her experience can be like a balm to any grief or trauma she may have experienced.

In our culture we find it very hard to talk about the dead, we tiptoe around anyone who may have recently lost a loved one, yet often that person is actually calling out to be asked about their loved one who recently passed over. There is a similarity between this experience and an abortion, when spoken about we are validating it as part of life's journey, part of the rich tapestry that makes us human and honours our capacity to love.

I give thanks to all the men, partners, and friends out there for supporting, loving and holding the women that go through an abortion. We are eternally grateful.

CHAPTER 9

Miscarriage

This book is about loss, loss of a small being that was growing in your womb and has now departed. The loss that I am focusing on is under the label of abortion, however if we look beyond that label to the simple fact that an abortion is the loss of a baby, we start to find similarities with other experiences of baby loss, such as miscarriage.

When a woman's body goes through a miscarriage, the physical aftermath can be very similar to an abortion. The body is suffering the same deep loss of a baby causing the hormones to go hay-wire and waves of emotions to run through the body. Yet the two experiences are very different from each other, one is an unintentional loss of a foetus and the other is an intentional loss. This difference has the potential to create a cavern between them, depending on each woman's thoughts on abortion. Whether you believe that both experiences can even be spoken about in the same sentence is totally subjective. If a woman is against abortion for whatever reason, then it is likely that these two experiences cannot be compared; however, many women will have gone through both and can therefore appreciate how similar the loss can be.

When spoken about, the general reaction is often completely different whether we say we had an abortion or a miscarriage. The first is often a reaction of shock, maybe judgement, and sadness. The second is sadness and often sympathy, despite both events causing a significant loss to the woman. Although each experience has its challenges and impact on a woman's life, there is no reason to treat one woman differently from the other. By looking at both miscarriage and abortion as baby loss, this nurtures a more compassionate non-judgemental view towards both experiences.

Jessica Zucker, a psychologist who specialises in reproductive and maternal mental health, has written book called *Miscarriage: A Memoir, A Movement* and speaks of both miscarriage and abortion.

> "Pregnancy loss is chock-full of what-ifs. It reinforces the idea that a person who has an abortion and a person who has a miscarriage are two different people. In reality, they are often one and the same, and just like they were able to make their own choices about their own bodies, they're capable of feeling a wide range of emotions in response to the many possible reproductive outcomes".[43]

If you have had a miscarriage and have come across this book, I welcome you with open arms into this space. The rituals, herbs, and tools that are woven throughout this book would be very helpful and suitable for any woman who has gone through a miscarriage and feels the need to gently honour their loss and heal their body.

Each and every ritual is perfectly adaptable to your own needs, and although you will see the word abortion everywhere, I hope this does not deter you from choosing to honour yourself as worthy of healing from your loss. If you are seeking help with rebalancing your body after a miscarriage, all the herbs that I have recommended in Chapter 3 are well-suited to assisting your body and womb recover.

There is a whole spectrum of herbs that can assist women who may be prone to miscarriages, I have not included them in this book however if you are called to seek ways that herbal medicine may be able to support your womb through another pregnancy, then I suggest you get in touch with a qualified medical herbalist who can support you on your journey.

EPILOGUE

Closing the circle

As I write these final words, I feel humbled to be part of an incredible ever evolving web of women who are changing the narrative around abortion. There were times when this book writing process brought up too much to go on; it has been a journey of deep inner work, demanding that I went into the depths of my own abortion, and work through any residing feelings of shame or grief. In those moments when I faltered on the path, I would hear of yet another woman's story about how she felt uncared for and unheard in the weeks and months after. These stories would pick me up off the floor and sit me down at my desk, inspiring me to continue this work.

At this time on earth, we are living through enormous change where the polarities of light and dark are becoming ever extreme. The patriarchy is still clinging on, clearly shown by countries continuing to clamp down on reproductive rights, despite intense and angry protests from women. Our work is not over. Aside from becoming involved politically with protests, how can we support those whose choice to end a pregnancy is one fraught with danger and risk?

Firstly we can create resources that are accessible for every woman who may need guidance on her journey. We can offer prayers to the women across the world who are going through dangerous procedures and finally we can remember the wisdom of herbs and their immense capacity to heal our bodies.

I close this space with a prayer to all women who are claiming their reproductive rights as their own, who are calling in the support from their sisters and who are reaching out to the women around them who need their help.

I offer my profound gratitude for each and every one of you who shared this journey with me. May we thrive as women in this world, and draw from the infinite well of strength that our ancestors are holding around us. May this give us courage to go on, to live our truths, and honour the wisdom of our beautiful selves.

Blessed be

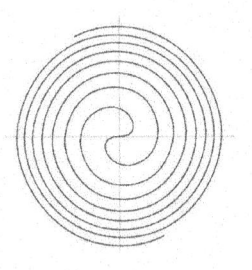

EPILOGUE 141

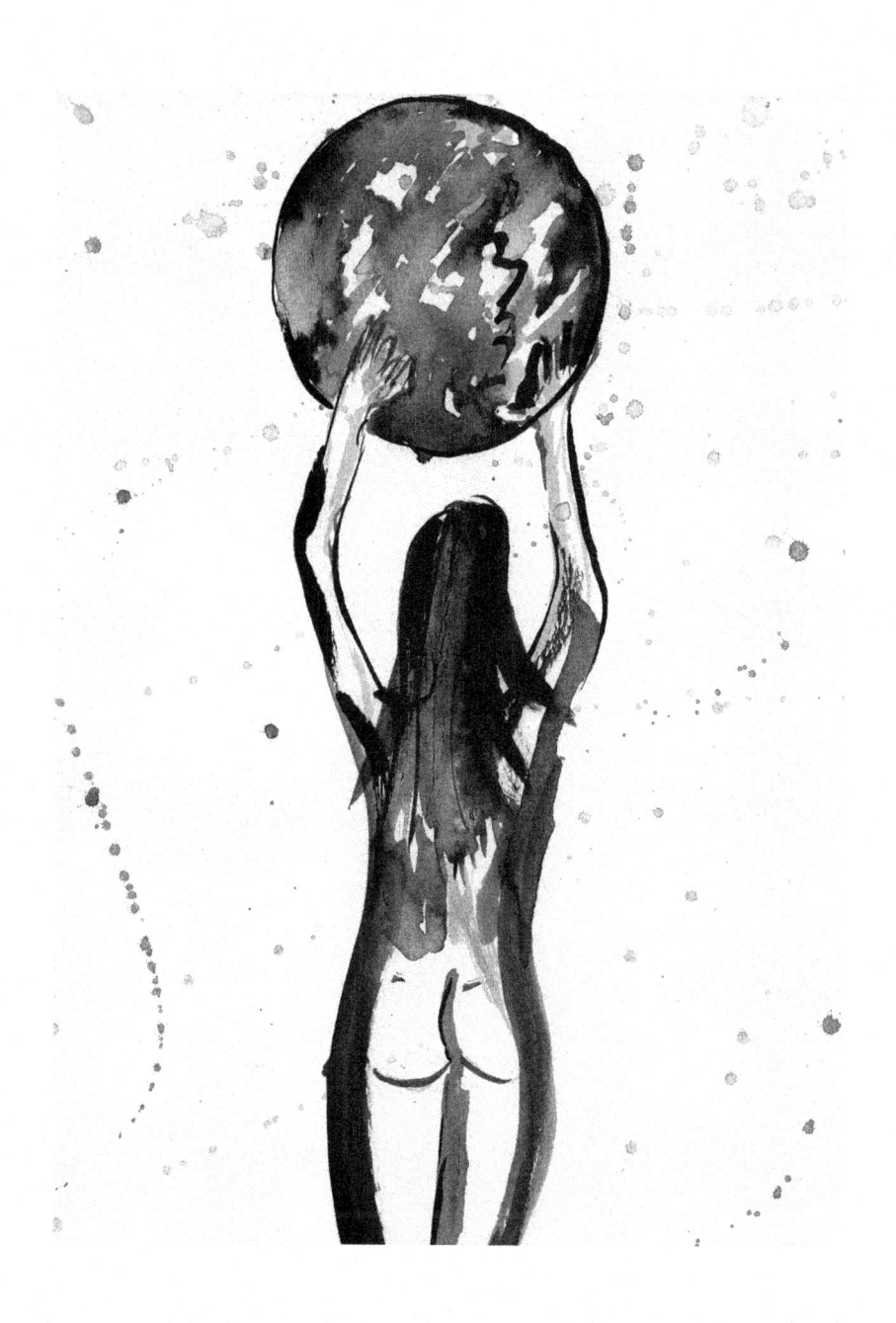

END NOTES

Chapter one
Choice of words

1. Etymonline. Etymology of abortion. Last accessed 2020. https://www.etymonline.com/search?q=abortion

Introduction

2. "Tami Lynn Kent, "The Vagina Whisperer", filmed at TEDx-Portland, last modified 10th July, 2018. [video]. YouTube. https://www.youtube.com/watch?v=rK_P0UmpYd8&t=3s&ab_channel=TEDxTalks
3. Brené Brown. *Daring Greatly: How the Courage to Be Vulnerable Transforms the Way We Live, Love, Parent, and Lead.* (USA: Penguin Random House, 2015), 96.
4. "Considering abortion?", British Pregnancy Advisory Service. Last accessed 10/5/2020, https://www.bpas.org/abortion-care/considering-abortion/
5. "Countries where abortion is illegal". Last accessed 10/5/2020. https://worldpopulationreview.com/country-rankings/countries-where-abortion-is-illegal.

END NOTES

6. Tami Lynn Kent, *The Wild Feminine*. (Atria Books/Beyond Words, New York, USA, 2011), 127.
7. Rosita Arvigo and Nadine Epstein, *Rainforest Home Remedies*, The Maya Way to Heal your Body & Replenish your Soul, (HarperCollins Publishers, 2001), 132.
8. Starhawk, The *Earth Path: Grounding Your Spirit in the Rhythms of Nature* (HarperOne, San Francisco, 2011), 309.
9. Lucy H. Pearce. *Burning Woman*. (Woman craft Publishing, 2016).
10. Brene Brown, *Daring Greatly: How the Courage to Be Vulnerable Transforms the Way We Live, Love, Parent, and Lead*. (USA: Penguin Random House, 2015). Paraphrased.
11. Claire Valentine, Breaking the Silence around abortion. 2020. https://www.papermag.com/abortion-scene-euphoria-cassie-2639652158.html?rebelltitem=8#rebelltitem8
12. Jeannine Parvati Baker, *Hygieia: A Woman's Herbal* (Self-published, San Francisco, USA, 1979).
13. Candace de Puy and Dana Dovitch, *The Healing Choice: Your guide to Emotional Recovery After an Abortion* (New York: Simon & Schuster, 1997), 119.
14. Merlin Stone, *Ancient Mirrors of Womanhood* (Beacon Press, Boston, USA 1984), 222.
15. 'Meaning of soul'. Cambridge Dictionary. 2020, https://dictionary.cambridge.org/dictionary/english/soul

Chapter two

Before an abortion

16. Walter Makichen, *Spirit Babes: How to Communicate with the Child You're Meant to Have*. (New York: Bantam Dell. Random House, 2005), 126.
17. Anonymous Testimony quoted in Jeannine Parvati Baker, *Hygieia: A Woman's Herbal*. (Self-published, San Francisco, USA, 1979), 202–203.
18. Anonymous account of a 'psychic abortion', quoted in Jeannine Parvati Baker, *Hygieia: A Woman's Herbal* (Self-published, San Francisco, USA, 1979), 202–203.
19. Nadine Epstein and Rosita Arvigo, *Spiritual Bathing* (Brattleboro, Vermont: Echo Point Books & Media, 2018).

Chapter three

Just after an abortion

20. Jackie Singer, *Birthrites, Rituals and Celebrations for the Child-bearing Years* (Permenant Publications, UK, 2009), 156.

21. Roslyne Sophia Breillat, The Pregnant Womb, The Trauma of Abortion, last accessed 2020. http://www.susunweed.com/herbal_ezine/July11/moon-magic.htm
22. Anna Druet, What to expect before, during and after abortion. Last accessed 2020. https://helloclue.com/articles/cycle-a-z/what-to-expect-before-during-and-after-an-abortion
23. https://www.healingherbs.co.uk/ Last accessed 2020.

Chapter four

Long-term after an abortion

24. Candace de Puy and Dana Dovitch, *The Healing Choice: Your guide to Emotional Recovery After an Abortion* (New York: Simon & Schuster, 1997), 179.
25. Francis Welller, *The Wild Edge of Sorrow* (Berkeley, California: North Atlantic Books, 2015), 99.
26. John O'Donohue, *To Bless the Space Between Us* (United States: Covergent Books, 2008), 157.
27. Brené Brown. *Daring Greatly: How the Courage to Be Vulnerable Transforms the Way We Live, Love, Parent, and Lead.* (USA: Penguin Random House, 2015), 68.
28. Weller, *The Wild Edge of Sorrow* (Berkeley, California: North Atlantic Books, 2015), 115.
29. Online Etymology Dictionary, bless(v), 2020. https://www.etymonline.com/word/bless
30. John O'Donohue, *To Bless the Space Between Us* (United States: Covergent Books, 2008), xiii.
31. Tami Lynn Kent, *The Wild Feminine.* (Atria Books/Beyond Words, New York, USA, 2011), 123.

Chapter five

Introduction on ritual

32. Weller, *The Wild Edge of Sorrow* (Berkeley, California: North Atlantic Books, 2015), 75.
33. Jackie Singer, *Birthrites, Rituals and Celebrations for the Child-bearing Years* (Permenant Publications, UK, 2009), 2.
34. John O'Donohue, *To Bless the Space Between Us* (United States: Covergent Books, 2008), xiv.

Rituals

35. 5 Scientifically proven reasons why the sea is good for you. Chiara Boracchi. Last accessed 2020. *https://www.lifegate.com/sea-benefits.*

Chapter six
Nutrition

36. Nutrition–womens extra needs. Last accessed 2020 https://www.betterhealth.vic.gov.au/health/healthyliving/nutrition-womens-extra-needs
37. Iron deficiency anemia. Last accessed 2020. https://www.nhs.uk/conditions/iron-deficiency-anaemia/
38. W R Phipps , M C Martini, J W Lampe, J L Slavin, M S Kurzer. "Effect of flax seed ingestion on the menstrual cycle." *J Clin Endocrinol Metab.* 1993 Nov;77(5):1215-9. doi: 10.1210/jcem.77.5.8077314. PMID: 8077314.
39. Jessica, Nourished by Nutrition, Seed Cycling for your hormones. Last accessed 2020. https://nourishedbynutrition.com/seed-cycling-for-hormone-balance/
40. Lara Briden, How to Lower Estrogen, last accessed 2020. https://www.larabriden.com/the-ups-and-downs-of-estrogen-part-2-estrogen-excess/
41. Sesame Seeds, last accessed 2020. http://www.whfoods.com/genpage.php?tname=foodspice&dbid=84

Chapter seven
Body and movement

42. Gaétan Chevalier, Stephen T. Sinatra, James L. Oschman, Karol Sokal, and Pawel Sokal. "Earthing: Health Implications of Reconnecting the Human Body to the Earth's Surface Electrons". *Journal of environmental and public health.* vol. 2012 (2012): 291541. doi:10.1155/2012/291541.

Chapter nine
Miscarriage

43. Jessica Zucker, The silent shame of women who have had an abortion and a miscarriage. Last accessed 2020. https://www.telegraph.co.uk/health-fitness/body/silent-shame-women-have-had-abortion-miscarriage/ end notes

RESOURCES

Healing

- Holistic Pelvic Care™—a gentle form of bodywork that includes inter-vaginal massage and pelvic floor bodywork to restore balance in a woman's pelvis. Originally pioneered by Tami Lynn Kent. Check online to find a local qualified practitioner.
- Arvigo Mayan Abdominal Massage Therapy—a form of pelvic massage that encourages the correct placement of the uterus within the pelvis, to help restore balance and health within the reproductive organs. www.arvigotherapy.com
- National Institute for Medical Herbalists—where to find a qualified medical herbalist. nimh.org.uk

Women's circles

- Red Tent. A directory that will guide you to the nearest Red Tent facilitator in your area. www.redtentdirectory.com
- Jewels Wingfield. Workshops for both women and men. Working with the themes of grief. https://jewelswingfield.com

Women's herbal wisdom and health

- Hygieia: A Woman's Herbal—Jeannine Parvati Baker
- Herbal Therapy for Women—Elisabeth Brooke
- The Women's Herbal Apothecary: 200 Natural Remedies for Healing, Hormone Balance, Beauty and Longevity, and Creating Calm.—JJ Pursell
- Wise Woman Herbal for the Childbearing Year—Susan Weed
- Adaptogens. Herbs for Strength, Stamina, and Stress Relief—David Winston, RH (AHG).
- Moon Time: A Guide to Celebrating Your Menstrual Cycle—Lucy H. Pearce
- The Healing Choice. Your Guide to Emotional Recovery After an Abortion—Candace de Puy Ph.d & Dana Dovitch Ph.d
- Wild Feminine: Finding Power, Spirit & Joy in the Female Body—Tami Lynn Kent.

Ceremony and ritual

- The Book of Ceremony: Shamanic Wisdom for Invoking the Sacred in Everyday Life—Sandra Ingerman
- Birthrites: Rituals and Celebrations for the Child-bearing Years—Jackie Singer
- The Wild Edge of Sorrow: Rituals of Renewal and the Sacred Work of Grief—Frances Weller.
- Healing Wisdom of Africa: Finding Life Purpose through Nature, Ritual and Community—Malidoma Patrice Some.
- Earth Wisdom: A Heartwarming Mix of the Spiritual, the Practical and the Proactive—Glennie Kindred.

Menstrual cycle wisdom

- Period Power: Harness Your Hormones and Get Your Cycle Working for You—Maisie Hill
- Wild Power: Discover the Magic of the Menstrual Cycle and Awaken the Feminine Path to Power—Alexandra Pope
- Red Moon: Understanding and Using the Creative, Sexual and Spiritual Gifts of the Menstrual Cycle—Miranda Gray

- Youtube. Wombdala talk—with Jewels Wingfield—spiritual teachings of womb cosmology for women. https://www.youtube.com/watch?v=jd_vjwDULmw&ab_channel=Jewels Wingfield
- The Wise Wound: Menstruation and Everywoman—Penelope Shuttle and Peter Redgrove.

Fertility awareness

- Taking Charge of your Fertility: The Definitive Guide to Natural Birth Control, Pregnancy Achievement and Reproductive Health—Toni Weschler.
- The Fifth Vital Sign: Master Your Cycle & Optimize your Health—Lisa Hendrickson-Jack.

Menopause

- Menopausal Years the Wise Woman Way—Susan Weed

Holistic nutrition

- Balance Your Hormones, Balance your Life: Achieving Optimal Health and Wellness through Ayurveda, Chinese Medicine, and Western Science—Dr. Claudia Welch. MSOM

Connecting to the earth

- Braiding Sweetgrass: Indigenous Wisdom, Scientific Knowledge and Teachings of the Plants—Robin Kimmerer
- If Women Rose Rooted: A Life-changing Journey to Authenticity and Belonging—Sharon Blackie
- The Sacred House: Where Women Weave Words Into The Earth—Carolyn Hillyer
- The Wild Flower Key. British Isles & N.W Europe.—Francis Rose.

Creative responses to pregnancy loss

- REPEAL. A dance piece that was filmed and created in India by Sophie Hutchinson and Linda Morris. It was made just before the referendum in Ireland 2018. https://vimeo.com/255284559

Physical healing

- 5Rhythms. A movement meditation practice created by Gabrielle Roth in the 1970's. Find you nearest group by heading the site—https://www.5rhythms.com/

Abortion support

- 03453008090 Marie Stopes Support Line (open 24hrs/7 days a week)
- BPAS (British Pregnancy Advisory Service). An informative site filled with useful information about different abortion options, what to expect and where to find support.

Makers and creators of beautiful products

- Bohobo Aromatherapies—gorgeous skincare, essential oil sprays and candles. www.bohoboaromatherapies.etsy.com
- Moonseed Rituals—delicious bathing salts and perfume oils. www.moonseedrituals.etsy.com
- LunaWisdom—menstrual moon charts for tracking your period and beautiful moon art postcards. www.lunawisdom.etsy.com

Crafting medicines

- Baldwins—A great source of glass jars, bottles, and tincture making equipment. www.baldwins.co.uk

Herbal dispensaries (UK)

- Baldwins. www.baldwins.co.uk
- Indigo Herbs. www.indigo-herbs.co.uk
- Fushi. www.fushi.co.uk
- Organic Herb Trading. www.organicherbtrading.com (for larger quantities of herbs only).

Wise women podcasts

- Medicine Stories by Amber Magnolia Hill. https://mythicmedicine.love/podcast/
- For the Wild. https://forthewild.world/

BIBLIOGRAPHY

Annwen. *Herbal Abortion, a woman's d.i.y. guide*. Leeds: Godhaven Ink, 2002.
Boland, Yasmin. *Moonology*. UK: Hay House, 2016.
Brooke, Elisabeth. *Herbal Therapy for Women*. London : Thorsons, 1992.
Cahill, Susan.Wise Women. USA: Norton, 1996.
De Bairacli Levy, Juliette. *Common Herbs for Natural Health*. Woodstock, New York: Ash Tree Publishing, 1997.
Epstein, Nadine and Rosita Arvigo. *Spiritual Bathing*. Vermont: Echo Point Books & Media, 2018.
Hillyer, Carolyn. *The Sacred House*. Lower Merripit Farm, Dartmoor: Seventh Wave Books, 2010.
Hopkins, John. What is the role of hormones during pregnancy?. https://www.hopkinsmedicine.org/health/conditions-and-diseases/staying-healthy-during-pregnancy/hormones-during-pregnancy. [accessed 5/09/2021].
Kerr, Sarah. "An Introduction to Ritual Healing". Filmed Calgary, Alberta. Video. Course no longer available, other related content available at: https://soulpassages.ca/programs/
Khalsa, Karta Purkh Singh and Michael Tierra. *The Way of Ayurvedic Herbs*. Delhi: Motilal Banarsidass, 2016.
Kimmerer, Robin. *Braiding Sweetgrass*. Canada: Milkweed Editions, 2013.

Lavender, Susan and Anna Franklin. *Herb Craft—A Guide to the Shamanic and Ritual Use of Herbs*. UK: Capall Bann Publishing, 1996.

Prakasha, Padma and Anaiya Aon. *Womb Wisdom, Awakening the Creative and Forgotten Powers of the Feminine*. Canada: Destiny Books, 2011.

Riddle, John M. *Contraception and Abortion from the Ancient World to the Renaissance*. First Harvard University Press, 1994.

Shuttle, Penelope and Peter Redgrove, The *WiseWound Menstruation and Everywoman*. New York, USA: Harper Collins Publishers, 1994.

Some, Malidoma Patrice. *Healing Wisdom of Africa: Finding Life Purpose through Nature, Ritual and Community*. New York: Tarcher/Putnam, 1998.

Starhawk, *The Earth Path*. New York: Harper Collins Publishers, 2005.

Weed, Susan S. Wise *Woman Herbal for the Childbearing Year*. Woodstock, New York: Ash Tree Publishing, 1986.

GLOSSARY

Adaptogenic—moderate the impacts of stress in the body by supporting the adrenals and endocrine system.
Alterative—used to be known as "blood cleansers", they strengthen and nourish the body, improving overall health.
Antidepressant—helps lessen a depressive state, improves mood.
Anti-haemorrhagic—reduces the risk of heavy bleeding, controls the loss of blood.
Anti-inflammatory—reduces inflammation in the body.
Antioxidant—reduces oxidation in the body. Protects cells from damage by free radicals.
Antiseptic—prevents infection, inhibits the unnecessary growth of microorganisms.
Antispasmodic—relieves and lessens muscle spasms.
Antiviral—works to combat and prevent viral infections.
Aphrodisiac—restore and increase sexual energy.
Astringent—have a drying effect on the body, contract the tissues therefore stopping excess flow of fluid, e.g. blood.
Cardiotonic—tones and strengthens the heart.
Carminative—assist the health of the digestive system through the removal of gas.

Circulatory tonic—assists with the overall circulation of blood in the body.
Clairvoyant—the ability to see beyond the realms of the physical world.
Demulcent—herbs that are mucilaginous and helps soothe and protect mucus membranes.
Diaphoretic—help the body to sweat, therefore release any toxins in the body.
Diuretic—herbs that can increase the flow of urine.
Emmenagogue—can provoke contractions in the uterus and bring on a period.
Endometrium—the inner layer of uterus, that which breaks down during a period.
Holistic—looking at something as a whole/from an overall perspective.
Hormone normaliser—restores balance to the hormones.
Nervine—restores normal function in the nervous system, reducing tension and anxiety.
Neuralgia—pain in the body from irritated or damaged nerve tissue.
Relaxant—relieves tension in the body, promotes general relaxation.
Sedative—promote sleep and encourage calm.
Solar plexus—an energy centre the sits just above your navel.
Soul—the spiritual/immortal aspect of humans, animals, plants. The essence of our beings.
Styptic—halt excess bleeding, often used for external wounds.
Tonic—increases overall strength and health in the body.
Uterine tonic—tones and strengthens the uterus, increases overall health of the reproductive system.
Uterus—the central reproductive organ in the female body.

ACKNOWLEDGEMENTS

Beginning with my dear family, who surrounded me with all the love and support I needed throughout this project. To my grandmothers, Elyn and Pauline, your presence and encouragement from behind the veil was immense, thank you. Pop, you would be so proud that I have written a book, know that I felt your love always from the other side. Mum, who gave me the space and encouragement to bring this project into creation, your generosity humbles me every day, thank you for holding the hearth with such love. My dear sister who so bravely lay next to me as I released my pregnancy all those years ago, those moments changed my life and you were an anchor of love throughout. My brothers, for being so tolerant of their sister who speaks about the moon and periods all the time. I love you all.

Geoffrey, le chemin de ce livre a commencé avec toi, chez toi. Merci pour ton encouragement depuis le début et pour ton amour pendant les moments difficiles, ton soutien a touché mon coeur. J'espere que cet petit livre noir dans les montagnes continue á aider plein des femmes qui a besoin du soutien des plantes. Bisous.

To Carole, BeautyPlantDreamer, my teacher. Thank you for joining the dots together right at the beginning of this journey, and having faith in me that this is what I had to do. Thank you for being a beacon of wisdom, for holding sacred space for such powerful transformations to occur, and for embodying the love of plants with so much joy. I am profoundly grateful to continue to be your student.

To the lovely team at Aeon, with a special mention to Melinda, thank you for being part of the movement to bring abortion to the light, and for having total faith in me that I can contribute to this important mission. To Jess, for the jumping in last minute to create a beautiful cover, thank you.

To the circle of dear sisters across the globe who have each been a pillar of support and love on this journey. You all inspire me more than you can ever know. **Chatty**, I offer such heartfelt thanks for your deep knowledge and wisdom on grief. Your suggestions helped me see grief from a wider perspective and offer ways of beauty to support women through this time. **Zen**, deep gratitude to you dearest sister for that bread we baked, and for your enthusiasm throughout, and offering your time to read these words. **Tara**, as a co-creator of our little women's circle you have been a beacon of womb support and love throughout, thank you for your creative insights and womb sharings. **Heather**, my magical plant sister, thank you for our deep sharings over the years, for your wisdom from the publishing side of things, and your support for this project. **Isabella**, womb sister of the moon, thank you for your love and for the journey of sisterhood that began that day when we walked back under the full moon. **Grace**, for sharing your story with me, and for all the joyous times when we lived together in Berlin. **Frink**, for the sea walks, swims, and cups of tea, thank you for being a reason to leave my house and venture out to share some of this beautiful coastal land. And finally, **Emma**, my dearest and oldest friend. Your courage and strength to live despite everything was remarkable and inspiring. Thank you for reminding me of how precious life is.

To all the other women who shared their abortion story with me, thank you for your courage and honesty. Each story gave me the strength to bring this work out into the world.

To the anonymous French women who started a movement across France giving hope to women who wanted an abortion another way. Thank you for putting your wisdom into a book and publishing what has long been buried. To the woman who truly began this journey with her tiny book, we may never meet but know that your bravery to put that information into words has changed my life and the lives of others, giving us hope that we hold the power in our hands.

ACKNOWLEDGEMENTS

To the plants; those who helped heal my body and continue to do so, those who called to be in this book, and to those many that exist outside of these pages but are there for each and every person should they call. Thank you for your wise and healing spirits. To the owls in our garden who even in daylight sounded their calls and sent me the courage and wisdom to go into the underworld and write this book. Thank you for holding space. To all the worlds of Grandmother Earth for reminding me of my roots every day, may I continue to be in service to your dream.

And finally to my ancestors, I created this book in honour of your guiding lights and wise ways. Your prayers run deep in my blood, may I continue to send out your blessings on this earth.

INDEX

abortion, xi, xvi
    act of honouring, xvi, xvii
    ancestral healing, xix–xx
    creative responses to, 149
    cultivating power to heal, xxii
    emotions after, xvii
    foetus, xii, xxvii–xxviii
    to heal after, xviii
    legal issues, xx–xxi
    Pill Method, The, xxvi
    power-from-within, xxiii
    shame, xix
    sharing of stories, xxiv
    soul, xxvi–xxviii
    support, 150
    types of, xxvi
    womb, xxi–xxii
abortion, after the, 43
    agnus castus, 61
    anxiety/depression/grief, 53–60
    catmint, 53
    cramp bark, 51–52
    cramps, 51–53

ectopic pregnancy, 45
emotionally triggering factors, 44
flower essences, 63–64
ginger, 51
hawthorn, 59–60
heavy bleeding, 47–51
herbal tea blends, 62–63
herbs, 46, 61
hormones, 60
lady's mantle, 50, 62
lavender, 58–59
lemon balm, 55
lemon verbena, 55
liquorice root, 56–57
motherwort, 52, 56
mugwort, 61
nettle, 47
oat straw, 53–54
raspberry leaf, 48–49
rose, 49, 54
rosemary, 57
self care, 64
shepherd's purse, 50–51

160 INDEX

skullcap, 54
St John's wort, 57–58
symptoms of complication, 45
tusli, 56
womb massage, 64–65
yarrow, 48
abortion, before the, 23
   basil, 36–37
   bleeding, 38
   chamomile, 32
   connecting to foetus, 24, 25–27
   flower baths, 38–42
   ginger, 36
   herbs to take, 30
   lemon balm, 30–31
   lime flowers, 32–33
   meditation, 28
   miscarriage, 38
   morning sickness, 35
   mugwort, 37–38
   need for communication with foetus, 24–25
   nervines, 30
   oat straw, 31
   passionflower, 34
   peppermint, 37
   practical ways to prepare, 29
   preparing womb for abortion, 37
   rose, 33–34
   skullcap, 35
   support system, 29–30
   visualisation exercise to say goodbye, 25–26
   ways to soothe body, 38
abortionem, xii
abortion, long term after, 67
   blessing, 75–76
   feminine living, 78
   grief, 72–74
   healing from abortion, 69
   herbal healing, 76
   menstrual cycle, 77, 81
   menstrual cycle and moon, 76–77
   moon, 82
   natural contraception, 83

   post-abortion symptoms, 70–71
   seasons of womb, 79
   sharing your experience, 69–70
   symptoms of depression, 68
   tracking menstrual cycle, 79–81
adaptogenic, 153
   herb, 56
agnus castus, 61
alterative, 153
ancestral healing, xix–xx
antidepressant, 153
anti-haemorrhagic, 153
anti-inflammatory, 153
antioxidant, 153
antiseptic, 153
antispasmodic, 153
antiviral, 153
anxiety/depression/grief, 53. *See also* abortion, after the
   hawthorn, 59–60
   lavender, 58–59
   lemon balm, 55
   lemon verbena, 55
   liquorice root, 56–57
   motherwort, 56
   oat straw, 53–54
   rose, 54
   rosemary, 57
   skullcap, 54
   St John's wort, 57–58
   tusli, 56
aphrodisiac, 153
astringent, 153

Baker, J. P., 26–27
baking ritual, 110–111. *See also* creative rituals
balm, 19–20. *See also* herbal medicine
   ingredients, 20
   method, 21
   usage, 20–21
basal body temperature (BBT), 80
base oil, 17, 112. *See also* infused oils; rituals
basil, 36–37. *See also* abortion, before the

INDEX

bathing ritual, 96–97, 113–114. *See also* rituals
BBT. *See* basal body temperature
beetroot and chocolate cake, 120. *See also* chocolate
   ingredients, 120
   method, 121
blessing, 75–76. *See also* abortion, long term after

cacao. *See* chocolate
cardiotonic, 153
carminative, 153
catmint, 53
cervical mucus (CM), 80
chamomile, 32, 113. *See also* abortion, before the; rituals
chocolate (cacao), 115, 119. *See also* magnesium
   cake and beetroot, 120–121
   divine hot, 119–120
circulatory tonic, 154
clairvoyant, 154
CM. *See* cervical mucus
connecting to earth, 149
contraception, natural, 83
courage, xxiv
cramp bark, 51–52
cramps, 51. *See also* abortion, after the
   catmint, 53
   cramp bark, 51–52
   ginger, 51
   motherwort, 52
creative rituals, 110. *See also* rituals
   baking ritual, 110–111
   bathing ritual, 113–114
   making womb bowl, 111–112
   ritual of release and self-love, 112–113
crystal, 113. *See also* rituals
cycle awareness method, 83

dance, 126
Dandelion, xxv
demulcent, 154

depression, 53. *See also* anxiety/depression/grief symptoms, 68
diaphoretic, 154
diuretic, 154
double boiler method, 19. *See also* infused oils

earth, 105
   connecting to earth, 149
   grounding to the earth, 126–127
   mixing your blood with earth, 106–107
ectopic pregnancy, 45. *See also* abortion, after the
elemental rituals, 104–105. *See also* rituals
   air, 104
   earth, 105
   fire, 104–105
   giving to waters, 107–109
   mixing your blood with earth, 106–107
   water, 105
emmenagogue, 154
endometrium, 154
essential oils, 112. *See also* rituals
essential vitamins and minerals, 116. *See also* nutrition

feminine living, 78
fertility awareness, 149
Fertility Awareness Method, 83
flax seeds, 122. *See also* hormones and seeds
flower baths, 38–39. *See also* abortion, before the
   flowers/plants to use, 39–41
   method, 41–42
   reasons to take, 39
flower essences, 63–64
foetus, xii, xxvii
foetus, connecting with, 24. *See also* abortion, before the
   meditation, 28

need for communication with foetus, 24–25
visualisation exercise to say goodbye, 25–26
ways of connecting, 25, 26–27

geranium, 113. *See also* rituals
ginger, 36, 51. *See also* abortion, before the
grief, 72. *See also* abortion, long term after; anxiety/depression/grief
   honouring, 131
   many sides of, 72–73
   ways to cope with, 73–74
grounding to the earth, 126–127

harmoniser, 57. *See also* liquorice root
hawthorn, 59–60, 133–134
healing. *See also* abortion, long term after
   ancestral, xix–xx
   from abortion, 69
   resources, 147
heavy bleeding, 47. *See also* abortion, after the
   lady's mantle, 50
   nettle, 47
   raspberry leaf, 48–49
   rose, 49
   shepherd's purse, 50–51
   yarrow, 48
herbal. *See also* herbal medicine
   abortion, 3
   decoction, 12–13
   dispensaries, 150
   healing, 76
   preparations, 9
   tea blends, 62–63
herbal medicine, 1
   balm, 19–21
   cultivating connection to plants, 5–6
   dosage, 15–16
   herbal decoction, 12–13
   herbal preparations, 9

   herbal teas, 9–12
   herbs and women, 2–3
   infused oils, 16–19
   meeting plants, 6–8
   for men, 133
   need for, 4–5
   OTC drugs, 5
   and pharmaceutical drugs, 4
   tinctures, 13–15
   working with herbs, 8–9
herbal rituals, 98. *See also* rituals
   mugwort smoke bundle, 98–100
   planting new life, 100–101
   vagina steam, 102–103
herbal teas/infusions, 9. *See also* herbal medicine
   blending herbs, 10–11
   dosage, 15
   herbs alleviating symptoms, 11–12
   herbs used, 10, 12
   preparation, 9–10
herbs, 46, 61, 113. *See also* rituals
   agnus castus, 61
   blending herbs, 10–11
   flower essences, 63–64
   herbal actions, 8
   for herbal decoction, 13
   herbal tea blends, 62–63
   herbs to support men, 132–133
   for infused oils, 17, 18
   lady's mantle, 62
   Latin name, 8
   mugwort, 61
   plant spirit, 8
   to take after abortion, 46, 61
   to take before abortion, 30
   used in herbal teas/infusions, 10, 12
   and women, 2–3
   working with herbs, 8–9
holistic, 154
honour, xvi
hormone, 60
   normaliser, 154
hormones and seeds, 121. *See also* nutrition

flax seeds, 122
pumpkin seeds, 122
seed cycling, 121
seed quantity, 122
sesame seeds, 122
sunflower seeds, 122

Indian goddess Kali, xxv
infused oils, 16. *See also* herbal medicine
    base oil, 17
    benefits of, 16
    double boiler method, 19
    fresh/dried herbs, 17
    herbs to use, 18
    preparation, 18
    requirements, 17
    sunlight method, 18
    usage, 16–17
infusions, 12. *See* herbal teas/infusions
iron, 116. *See also* nutrition
    importance, 116–117
    nettle miso broth, 117–118
    sources of, 116

jasmine, 113. *See also* rituals
journaling, 109. *See also* writing rituals

lady's mantle, 50, 62
lavender, 58–59
lemon
    balm, 30–31, 55. *See also* abortion, before the
    verbena, 55
letter of forgiveness, 109–110. *See also* writing rituals
letter writing, 95–96. *See also* rituals
life and death, xxiv–xxv
lime flowers, 32–33. *See also* abortion, before the
linseeds. *See* flax seeds
liquorice root, 56–57

magnesium, 118–119. *See also* chocolate; nutrition
Makichen, W., 24

medicines, crafting, 150
men, 129
    hawthorn, 133–134
    herbal medicine, 133
    herbs to support men, 132–133
    nettle, 134
    oat straw, 135
    rosemary, 134
    sage, 134
    skullcap, 135
    support for, 130
    supporting themselves, 130–132
    to support woman, 135–136
    taking herbs, 133
menopause, 149
menstrual cycle, 81. *See also* abortion, long term after
    benefits to understanding, 77
    and moon, 76–77
    resources, 148–149
    tracking menstrual cycle, 79–81
mifepristone, xxvi
miscarriage, 38, 137–138. *See also* abortion, before the
misoprostol, xxvi
moon, 82
    menstrual cycle and, 76–77
    tinctures, 15
    ways to connect to, 82
morning sickness, 35. *See also* abortion, before the
motherwort, 52, 56, 113. *See also* rituals
mugwort, 37–38, 61. *See also* abortion, before the
    smoke bundle, 98–100. *See also* herbal rituals

nervines, 30, 154. *See also* abortion, before the
nettle, 47, 134
nettle miso broth, 117–118. *See also* iron
    ingredients, 118
    method, 118
neuralgia, 154

INDEX

nutrition, 115
    chocolate, 115, 119–121
    essential vitamins and minerals, 116
    hormones and seeds, 121–122
    iron, 116–117
    magnesium, 118–119
    nettle miso broth, 117–118
    resources, 149
    supplements, 117

oat straw, 31, 53–54, 135. *See also* abortion, before the
oestrogen, 60
ovarian energy, xxi
over the counter drugs, 5
oxytocin, 60

passionflower, 34. *See also* abortion, before the
peppermint, 37. *See also* abortion, before the
Period Cake, The. *See* beetroot and chocolate cake
periods. *See* menstrual cycle
physical healing, 150
Pill Method, The, xxvi, 116–117
plants. *See also* herbal rituals
    cultivating connection to, 5–6
    meeting plants, 6–8
    planting new life, 100–101
post-abortion physical and emotional symptoms, 70–71. *See also* abortion, long term after
power-from-within, xxiii
pregnancy, ending. *See* abortion
pregnancy loss. *See* abortion
premenstrual tension (PMT), xxii
progesterone, 60
pumpkin seeds, 122. *See also* hormones and seeds

raspberry leaf, 48–49
relaxant, 154
release and self-love, 112–113. *See also* creative rituals

resources, 147
    abortion support, 150
    ceremony and ritual, 148
    connecting to the earth, 149
    crafting medicines, 150
    creative responses to pregnancy loss, 149
    fertility awareness, 149
    healing, 147
    herbal dispensaries, 150
    holistic nutrition, 149
    makers and creators of beautiful products, 150
    menopause, 149
    menstrual cycle wisdom, 148–149
    physical healing, 150
    wise women podcasts, 150
    women's circles, 147
    women's herbal wisdom and health, 148
rituals, 85, 94
    and abortion, 86–87
    before an abortion, 94
    after an abortion, 97–98
    aspects of, 91–92
    author experience, 93–94
    baking ritual, 110–111
    bathing ritual, 96–97, 113–114
    creating your own rituals, 90–91
    creative rituals, 110
    elemental rituals, 104–105
    example of simple, 92–93
    giving to waters, 107–109
    herbal rituals, 98
    journaling, 109
    lanting new life, 100–101
    letter of forgiveness, 109–110
    making womb bowl, 111–112
    for men, 132
    mixing blood with earth, 106–107
    need for ritual after abortion, 87
    passing through threshold, 87–89
    of release and self-love, 112–113
    resources, 148
    ugwort smoke bundle, 98–100
    vagina steam, 102–103

writing rituals, 95–96, 109
rose, 33–34, 49, 54. *See also* abortion, before the; rituals
    petals, 113
rosemary, 57, 134

sage, 134
salts, 112. *See also* rituals
sedative, 154
seed. *See also* hormones and seeds
    cycling, 121
    quantity, 122
self care, 64. *See also* abortion, after the
serotonin, 119
sesame seeds, 122. *See also* hormones and seeds
shame, xix
shepherd's purse, 50–51
skullcap, 35, 54, 135. *See also* abortion, before the
solar plexus, 154
soul, xxvi–xxvii, 154
St John's wort, 57–58
styptic, 154
sunflower seeds, 122. *See also* hormones and seeds
sunlight method, 18. *See also* infused oils
supplements, 117. *See also* nutrition
sweet orange, 113. *See also* rituals

threshold, 87–89. *See also* rituals
tinctures, 13. *See also* herbal medicine
    benefits of, 14
    dosage, 15–16
    gratitude for plants, 15
    and moon, 15
    need for, 13–14

    preparation, 14–15
tonic, 154
    cardiotonic, 153
    circulatory tonic, 154
    uterine tonic, 154
tusli, 56
two-pill method, 47. *See also* abortion, after the

uterine tonic, 154
uterus, 154

vagina steam, 102. *See also* herbal rituals
    benefits of, 102
    method, 103
    when not to have, 102
voice, 127–128

wise women podcasts, 150
womb, xxi–xxii
    bowl, 111–112
    massage, 64–65
    preparing womb for abortion, 37
    seasons of womb, 79
women's
    circles, 147
    herbal wisdom and health, 148
    voices, 127
writing rituals, 109. *See also* rituals
    journaling, 109
    letter of forgiveness, 109–110

yarrow, 48
yoga, 124–125

Zucker, J., 138